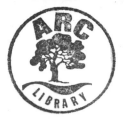

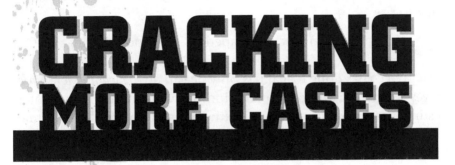

"No one individual is more responsible for opening the door of science and having its sunlight shine in American courtrooms than Dr. Henry Lee. . . . The cases he describes in this book are a testament not only to the lingering ignorance of the past, but to a clear vision of the extremely promising future. . . . If we could assemble all of the participants in the criminal justice system in a gigantic stadium—judges, prosecutors, police, victims, and innocent defendants—they would all rise and give Henry Lee a standing ovation. I would be the first to rise."

—Connecticut Superior Court Judge Charles D. Gill

"Henry Lee has done it again as only he can do. *Cracking More Cases* gives us his insight and explanation of five memorable and interesting cases in an informative, instructive, and very readable format. Forensic science can aid in apprehending the guilty and exonerating the innocent, and nobody is better at it than Dr. Henry Lee."

—Haskell M. Pitluck
Illinois Circuit Court Judge (retired)
past president of the American Academy of Forensic Sciences

"*Cracking Cases* is required reading for all my Homicide Detectives and Crime Scene Personnel. *Cracking More Cases* will also be required reading. There is so much to learn from Dr. Henry Lee's experiences."

—Sheriff Harry Lee
Jefferson Parish, Louisiana

"Dr. Lee's most recent real-life crime thriller takes you to the crime scene like no TV show ever will—with truth and reality. He's the best and this book proves it again."

—Mary Galvin, State's Attorney for Milford, Connecticut,
and frequent Crime Scene Visitor

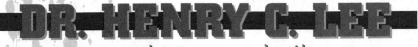

DR. HENRY C. LEE

with **thomas w. o'neil**

CRACKING MORE CASES

THE FORENSIC SCIENCE OF SOLVING CRIMES

the michael skakel–martha moxley case
the jonbenet ramsey case and many more!

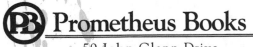

Prometheus Books

59 John Glenn Drive
Amherst, New York 14228-2197

Published 2004 by Prometheus Books

Inquiries should be addressed to
Prometheus Books
59 John Glenn Drive
Amherst, New York 14228–2197
VOICE: 716–691–0133, ext. 207
FAX: 716–564–2711
WWW.PROMETHEUSBOOKS.COM

08 07 06 05 04   5 4 3 2 1

Library of Congress Cataloging-in-Publication Data

Lee, Henry C.
    Cracking more cases : the forensic science of solving crimes / Henry C. Lee with Thomas W. O'Neil.
        p. cm.
    Includes bibliographical references and index.
    ISBN 1–59102–199–5 (hardcover : alk. paper)
    1. Murder—Investigation—Case studies. 2. Forensic sciences—Case studies. 3. Evidence, Criminal. 4. Criminal investigation—Case studies. I. O'Neil, Thomas. II. Title.

HV8079.H6L44 2004
363.25'9523—dc22

2004007099

Printed in Canada on acid-free paper

To Mrs. An-Fu Lee
mother and educator
and our deep gratitude
to all of the others who
have helped us

CONTENTS

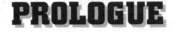

PROLOGUE

Time is the wisest counselor.

—Ancient Chinese proverb

The words with which I begin this book relate very directly to forensic science in today's world. Technological breakthroughs achieved in the last decade have meant that police investigators have been able to reopen and solve many very old, "cold" cases. These are crimes that have vexed many fine police detectives who, in earlier times, were unable to find that one key link in a chain of evidence that meant the guilty would have been successfully prosecuted, while the innocent could have been set free. Two of the five cases covered in this book, both murders in Connecticut, became very cold cases: the July 16, 1973, murder of Concetta "Penney" Serra in a New Haven parking garage and the October 30, 1975, slaying of Martha Moxley, adjacent to her home in Greenwich.

Both of these murders went unsolved for decades. Both of these cases are today solved, and the accused parties have been convicted. And both cases, quite naturally, are under judicial appeal, and until those reviews have been completed, the possibility exists that either conviction or both may be overturned. If that happens, each case will, in all probability, be retried. However, the governing investigative facts that helped solve these two murders stand for themselves and, thus, are being presented in this book. All five cases covered here present examples of the critical role that forensic evidence plays not only in extablishing the manner and cause of death, but also in providing important investigative leads.

I am constantly asked what cases am I presently working on, by my colleagues, friends, and members of the general public whom I meet in my travels, or at lectures I give at meetings and dinners. Of course, I try to respond to any and all questions, though I cannot directly comment on most of those current cases that are still active, sometimes due to a specific judicial gag order. All of these questions from a broad range of American citizens have made me, in turn, ask myself why there seems to be such an increase in interest in forensic investigations and the science of solving crimes. It has reached a point where it seems impossible to turn on a television set at any time of the day or night and not find a program about forensic investigators and their attempts to solve complicated crimes. This has made me reflect on this rapidly growing trend, and I've come up with one or two possible hypotheses on all of this. First, Americans today seem to genuinely want to know who has committed a crime. This feeling is time-honored and has often been called "a thirst for justice." This tendency has only been heightened by the events of September 11, 2001, and our country's unfinished prosecution of the terrorists who committed those heinous acts. Other sensational cases, including the Lindbergh baby kidnapping-murder, the Dr. Sam Sheppard case, the assassination of President Kennedy, and the 1994 murders of Nicole Brown Simpson and Ron Goldman, have also stirred deep curiosity and feelings. The second major factor driving public interest in these forensic stories, it seems to me, is the intellectual challenge presented by so many cases, a trend accelerated by the scientific breakthroughs achieved with new high-tech equipment. People seem to like to follow the investigators as they move toward the solution of a murder or kidnapping. Eventually, a case is solved through the forensic evidence, and what had appeared to be an impossible web of facts can be boiled down to a few simple conclusions.

On the one hand, I am happy that Americans, including many young students, have become so interested in the forensic science field and care so much about solving crimes through scientific evidence. I do not consider this interest as morbid, especially in light of the awful acts that one human being is capable of inflicting on a fellow mortal. At times, though, I have to shake my head in disbelief when I discover what has happened. The news media are only doing their jobs when they publicize these crimes, although media excesses have become an increasing problem for police investigators and prosecutors. After JonBenet Ramsey's little body was discovered in the basement of her home, the day after Christmas in 1996, the media's coverage blazed like a firestorm, and their abuses of the privileges afforded by the First Amendment seriously impeded that investigation. I only hope that the unethical behaviors displayed by a few in the media in that case, as discussed in this book, represent a nadir in press, television, and radio misconduct and that such abuses will never happen again. While I am on the subject of what is written and broadcast about criminal cases, let me add a thought on the amount of space devoted to the five cases in this book. Three of the cases that appear in this book have commanded much more attention from me than the other two. This is due to the cases' respective complexity and to the length of time involved in the investigation of each of these five cases.

I do not want to appear negative in my comments about the press concerning the cases presented in this book, the third of its kind I have authored. The news media have often provided critical assistance to investigators. And, though the Fourth Estate is independent, when investigators and responsible journalists have worked together for the common good, criminals are captured, convicted, and sent to jail at a much higher rate than usual. This is fundamental to our American way of life. Going back to the crime waves that swept across Depression America, when a paper printed the photo of a wanted man, the chances of his capture skyrocketed. Of course, this kind of news coverage also drove up circulation figures and showed the general public, long skeptical of the press, that the media have a crucial and positive role to play in our everyday lives.

There are other difficult facts and conclusions that one can draw from the five cases in this book. Investigators, being human, can make mistakes. This fact is not a source of pleasure for me to contemplate, let alone discuss in this volume. I started out my professional career in Taiwan as a cop in uniform. I know firsthand the difficulties confronting officers on the beat and how these complexities increase exponentially as one moves ahead in rank and responsibility. And for every mistake made by an officer, there are many more instances of conscientious police professionals doing their work extremely well. In the Penney Serra case, I have to draw attention to a fundamental mistake that the lead investigator made in the first few months that followed this murder and the tunnel vision that quickly developed. Yet this case would never have been solved were it not for the meticulous records and reports authored by the investigative team. When I was first asked to examine this case, I also had the use of a battery of excellent crime scene photos, taken by Sgt. Vincent Perricone, Det. Roy Olson, Officer Robert Fonteyn, and, of course, Ken Zercie, who at the time was a detective assigned to identification. Ken later became a student of mine. In 1989 he joined the State Police Forensic Science Laboratory and has now been promoted to assistant director of the lab. This visual record was critical to my being able to piece together a satisfactory reconstruction of the events that played out in the Penney Serra murder. My hat is off to these professionals and to the many other fine police officers who helped to solve this and many other heinous crimes.

Forensic articles of evidence should speak for themselves. I truly cannot overemphasize this point. Whenever I am approached by a prosecution or defense team, I quickly make clear that I will, to the best of my ability, find the scientific facts in a case, no matter where these facts take me and whether or not these facts please or displease those who have sought out my advice and expertise. Put another way, all of this work is not about personalities, or about whether a certain individual is an old friend of mine, or whether he's been an adversary. Being human, I often find myself meeting new and interesting people while I am working on a particular case, individuals with whom I strike up a genuine friendship. I remember flying to Bosnia on a chartered flight in the late nineties to investigate the mass grave sites left there and in Croatia after years of atrocities. I was making this trip at the invitation of Americare. During the long flight, a very pleasant young man introduced himself to me as Steven Skakel, who was nine the night that Martha Moxley was murdered next to his family's home. We both chuckled when Steven quickly cleared up the fact that he was not either of the Skakel brothers I had for years been investigating. The two of us struck up a friendship. Steven's aunt Ethel was married to the late senator Robert F. Kennedy, and I had assisted another Kennedy cousin, William Kennedy Smith, in his defending himself against a rape charge in the early nineties. This is not about personalities. It is about the forensic evidence and how this leads us all to the truth.

Just as with Steven Skakel, I have become close friends with many individuals as I do my work. Sometimes a person who is a friend stands out as particularly heroic to me. Alex Hunter, who left public service as a result of a very difficult decision he made in the JonBenet Ramsey case, is one such hero. I would like to complete my prologue to this book on that note. Mr. Hunter, who remains a good friend, presented a profile in courage to me, at least, when he saw his highly successful twenty-eight-year career as the Boulder County prosecutor end because he chose to do the right thing. Alex is not the only friend of mine who has risen above his own personal goals to perform a noble act, sometimes to his or her own profound detriment. There are others. I want to take this opportunity to thank them for their service to our legal and law enforcement communities. This is what drives me to work as hard as I can. I hope that this desire to persevere for the truth, no matter how long it takes others and me, is what comes across in the cases that we present in this book.

CHAPTER ONE

THE CONCETTA "PENNEY" SERRA CASE

A FATHER'S QUEST

"*PENNEY SERRA
MURDERED IN TEMPLE
STREET GARAGE,
Downtown, New Haven on
July 16, 1973 (DAYTIME).
To date, KILLER STILL IN
NEW HAVEN AREA!
Paid for by John Serra*"

—Text of an advertisement that appeared in
the *New Haven Register*, on
Saturday, July 16, 1988, fifteenth anniversary
of Penney Serra's murder.

In a 1988 newspaper interview with Joseph Brady of the *New Haven Register*, I mentioned that I thought that the 1973 Penney Serra murder could someday be solved due to the rapid advances taking place in the forensic science field.[1] The case was already fifteen years old, and its investigation seemed to be badly stymied. But, by then, I had witnessed the dramatic advances that were made in forensic serology, particularly developments pertaining to DNA. The Serra murder had left behind a trail of blood evidence. But, with the blood-grouping technology available in the early seventies, the forensic lab could determine only that the victim's blood was type A and that her assailant's was type O. These two blood types are both quite common, particularly type O (approximately 46 percent of the world's population is type O), so that finding a suspect with that type of blood would not represent a telling piece of evidence. When it came time for the prosecution to take its case to a jury trial, blood typing of that era helped more to rule out a particular defendant, rather than to individualize the person who had actually committed the crime. In addition to the blood evidence in this case, the investigator also discovered a number of partial unidentified fingerprints at the crime scene. But since there was no ready match for any of these prints, these pieces of evidence could not, in and of themselves, drive the case to a successful solution. Finally, the time-honored trust that the police and the public hold for eyewitness accounts further clouded this case and contributed to its failure to develop. This problem was only exacerbated when it became known that one young witness had been inhaling marijuana a few minutes before he saw a man chasing a young woman through the crime scene. All of these factors added up to the case's becoming very old and very cold. But, in 1994, the combination of new forensic techniques and the chance arrest of a man for battering his fiancée changed everything for the Serra case, moving the case toward its ultimate and successful prosecution.

In mid-July of 1973, Concetta "Penney" Serra worked as a dental assistant in an office on Chapel Street in the heart of New Haven's bustling downtown area. An attractive young woman, Penney, at twenty-one, was very responsible for her age, especially since she had become the family's homemaker ten years earlier when her mother had passed away. This meant that Penney, who was born on March 2, 1952, helped raise her younger sibling, Rosemary, five years her junior. The older sister also had dinner waiting for John Serra when he returned home from running his business, an auto repair shop located a quarter of a mile or so from New Haven's commercial harborfront on Long Island Sound. Quite bright, Penney also mastered her father's bookkeeping duties and helped manage his business. Thus, she had blossomed into a generous and mature young woman, well beyond someone of her limited life experience.

Though she was very intelligent, Penney had never sparkled academically at Wilbur Cross High School, where she'd graduated on June 25, 1971. In her high school yearbook, *The Crossroads*, Penney lists only a few extracurricular activities, such as serving on her junior and senior prom committees. Each of the four hundred or so graduates chose a verse or a saying to appear under his or her graduation photo, and Penney's selection seems particularly tragic today: "a laughing heart and merry spirit." She listed her favorite hobby as reading, and for her future she put only, "College." Her picture appears only once in the publication.[2] Penney Serra seemed to prefer to blend in with the other sixteen hundred students at the largely white school, one that, like New Haven itself, was dominated by her fellow Italian Americans. She concentrated, instead, on her family life and her growing circle of friends. Penney had a good, quick sense of humor and was known for her loyalty to those close to her. Her brunette hair was longish, extending down to just below her shoulders, customary for those times, hair that was parted in the middle, just above her forehead, showing her direct, clear brown eyes. Like almost all of her schoolmates, Penney loved the era's rock 'n' roll music that seemed to flourish in the sixties, and she liked to go out to clubs where she and her friends could dance. Penney also enjoyed driving the Serra family cars, which were kept in impeccable condition by her father. Driving away from the family's neat and comfortable home on Huntington Avenue in one of New Haven's shoreline sections, called the Annex, Penney could quickly find herself cruising along the Connecticut Turnpike. She could either head east, toward Boston, a two-and-a-half-hour drive, or she could drive west, toward New York City, only an hour and a half away.

On the hot and muggy morning of Friday, July 16, 1973, Penney

Serra's future seemed to beckon to her. True, her college plans had been shelved, at least for the time being. Instead, Penney was making a living in the dental field, work that she seemed to enjoy, especially since her duties put her in contact with a wide variety of people. Though she could be quite feisty on occasion, Penney liked people and drew satisfaction from helping her patients get through their onerous visits to the dentist. Penney's maturity seemed in sharp contrast to most of the thousands of college students who studied at one of New Haven's six institutions of higher learning, including Yale. It was not at all surprising, then, that Penney became engaged for a time to Philip DeLieto, an attractive man seven years older than she who was distantly related to New Haven's chief of police, Biagio "Ben" DiLieto. Penney's boyfriend worked at his family's luncheonette in the downtown business area about a mile from her own workplace. But, as time wore on, Phil and Penney found themselves frequently quarreling, so much so that, at Penney's insistence, the couple became unengaged, though they continued to see one another and to take trips together until the day Penney was murdered. Phil DeLieto was the first of the three men who would become early prime suspects in her murder. However, the investigative preoccupation with DeLieto or the other early suspects did not cost the case valuable years, since the deus ex machina that eventually led to the solving of the Penney Serra murder did not exist then and would not exist for decades.

The passage of time can create interesting contrasts. In 1960 I was promoted to the rank of captain on the Taiwan national police force and was only just then formulating plans for my wife, Margaret, and me to come to the United States to further our studies. I arrived in New York City in 1965. During the first ten years, I worked at the New York University Medical Center as a research assistant and attended classes at night. I also waited on tables at a Chinese restaurant and taught Kung Fu and karate on weekends to support my family and myself. In 1975 I received my PhD in Biochemistry from New York University, specializing in molecular biology, and accepted an offer from the University of New Haven to become an assistant professor and to create a forensic science program. After we arrived in New Haven in 1975, I do not precisely remember the first time I ever heard of the Serra murder. But I do know, as I once testified in court, I would spend a tremendous amount of my time and energy on this case, enough to make it all feel like a lifetime.

The Penney Serra murder eventually became a very cold case. The efforts of her father, John Serra, and the advertisements taken out in the local papers by him helped to keep the case in the public mind. John Serra would later befriend me. After I became director of the Connecticut State Police Forensic Science Laboratory, John Serra visited me a number of times in my Meriden office to press me in any way he could to discover who had so cruelly taken the life of his beautiful daughter. Yet, even with these personal visits and the thousands of dollars that Mr. Serra spent on newspaper ads over the course of the twenty-five years before his own death, the murder of Penney Serra had become a crime that seemed to defy solution. Part of the problem was due to the rudimentary nature of blood evidence in 1973, an obstacle that eventually would be resolved by breakthroughs and advances in DNA technology and the enhancement of fingerprints. Another partial cause for the years it took to solve this crime was the initial work done by the New Haven police force itself. And, finally, the fact that an early primary suspect was distantly related to the city's chief of police fueled a great deal of public skepticism about how and why the crime had not yet been solved. This public reaction in 1973 would even be shared by one of the country's most illustrious television newsmagazine shows, a 1988 production that cast even more shadowy suspicions over the murder, shrouding further the ultimate identity of Penney Serra's killer.

As with the solving of many cold cases, it took teamwork and a stroke of luck to finally link a suspect to the investigation. This good fortune was, ironically, driven in large part by the killer's own behaviors, the same behavior patterns that had originally led to Penney Serra's terrible and untimely death in 1973. And, unlike the 1975 murder of Martha Moxley, covered in the next chapter, this murderer was not an individual any logical person who knew Penney Serra ever would have been able to identify. Here is how this 1973 case was eventually solved.

THE FACTS OF THE CASE

In 1973 New Haven was changing rapidly, perhaps even more so than the rest of America. With the war in Vietnam winding down, city planners were ambitiously putting in place strategies for attracting back to the central urban areas the thousands of former residents who had moved out into the suburbs during the years of prosperity following World War II. Large tracts of New Haven's inner-city housing were pulled down to make way for the freeways and the other roadways that would make it convenient and simple for shoppers and theatergoers to use the city's stores and entertainment venues. Huge, multilevel parking garages were built in and around New Haven's extensive medical facilities, its shopping mall, and the city's theaters. One of these additions was the gray Temple Street Garage.

Penney Serra had decided to take a day off on Friday, July 16. She wanted to pay some bills and run some other errands, so she would need to use the family car, her father's 1971, two-door, blue Buick Electra 225. Perhaps she would stop by the luncheonette where her boyfriend and ex-fiancé, Phil DeLieto, worked the counter on busy weekdays. Though the couple had recently decided to drop their plans to get married, Penney and Phil still enjoyed an on-again, off-again romance. The previous weekend the two had traveled down to the Rhode Island beaches with friends and spent Saturday night there.

On that Friday, July 16, Penney's younger sister, Rosemary, also had plans for the Buick, so the two sisters squabbled over who would get to use the family car. Not surprisingly, the older sister won the argument. Penney left the house around 11:00 AM. On her way to downtown New Haven, Penney dropped by her father's auto garage, where she did the bookkeeping, and visited briefly. She pulled out around 11:30 AM. This was the last time that any member of her family would ever see Penney Serra alive.

Very little is known about Penney Serra's activities and whereabouts for the next hour and a quarter or so. She had plans, she'd told her father, to buy some furniture on sale at the Edward Malley's department store for her family's home.[3] Perhaps she spent some moments across the street from Malley's, in New Haven's air-conditioned new mall, at its Macy's department store, or outside, window-shopping and walking past the shops and boutiques on Chapel Street, the city's upscale retail district. Since this was the heart of the summer, there would be only a smattering of Yale students downtown. In the Buick again, Penney drove into the Frontage Road entrance of the Temple Street Garage at 12:42 PM and parked the car on the ninth level. At 12:43 PM, a minute after Penney Serra had pulled into the facility, another auto entered the garage from the George Street

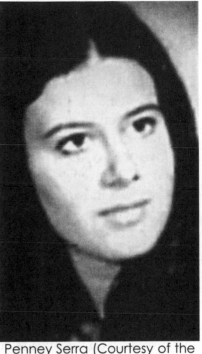

Penney Serra (Courtesy of the New Haven Register)

entrance, the one facing north. In all probability, that driver was the very next person Penney Serra talked to, someone who killed her, just before 1:00 PM, after frantically chasing her by foot through several levels of the parking garage. This murderer's identity remained a deep secret for more than twenty-five years, and his motive to this day is shrouded in mystery.

THE INVESTIGATION OF THE CASE

Shortly after 1:00 PM on Friday, July 16, Mike Lundgren* (I will be using asterisks to denote pseudonyms throughout the book), an employee for the New Haven Parking Authority at the Temple Street Garage, returned from his lunch break. Lundgren was walking through the tenth and top level of the garage when he saw something lying at the base of a stairwell leading up to the top of the building's elevator shaft. Advancing to the corner stairwell, Lundgren saw the body of a young woman lying in a fetal position on the bottom two steps of the stairwell, her head pointing downward toward the base of the stairs. She wore no shoes, and the soles of her feet appeared soiled. The woman's blue dress was drenched with blood, and Lundgren immediately determined that she was dead. At that time, a parked Jeep was the only vehicle at the top level. The employee called the police, and within minutes two patrol cars arrived at the scene. After making the call to police, the garage employee was moving down from the tenth to the ninth level of the garage when he saw what appeared to be a brown wig. Later, this was shown to police, who seized it as evidence.

Police investigators quickly cordoned off the crime scene, and, as their numbers grew, they rapidly fanned out to investigate the lower levels of the garage. On the eighth level, in section A, police found an unlocked 1971 blue Buick Electra 225 parked at an erratic angle. Investigating the auto, police found quantities of a reddish, bloodlike substance on the outside door handle and door surfaces, on the car's steering shaft, on the floor of the driver's side, and on the aluminum trim both inside and outside the car. By 1:30 PM the department's photographer was taking black-and-white shots of the car and the body on the tenth level, as well as of other evidence. Using the car's Connecticut license plate numbers, police determined that the owner was John Serra of Huntington Avenue. On the car's front seat, investigators also found a pair of women's clogs and a brown purse containing, among other personal items, a wallet with $14.75. Also inside the wallet was the Connecticut driver's license of Concetta Serra. On the passenger seat, they found a pair of gold-rimmed glasses and a Temple Street Garage parking ticket marked with a 12:42 time of entry for that day. Police also found a pair of unopened envelopes behind the vehicle's driver's-side sun visor containing dental invoices for Martin Cooratal,* a patient at the office where Penney Serra worked. Looking at the auto's floor behind the driver's seat, police found more reddish, bloodlike stains on the vehicle's blue interior carpeting and on a pink Rite Aid tissue box.

Several tissues had been removed from the box, and police found reddish, bloodlike smears on it as well. On the same flooring, police came upon a colored rag, similar to those used by auto mechanics, and a white envelope that bore reddish stains.

Police also found a trail of drops and spatters leading away from the Buick and toward the stairwell extending upward toward the ninth and tenth levels. This trail led police to the northwest-corner stairwell where Penney Serra's body lay still. Now led by Nicholas Pastore, a chief inspector from the New Haven Police Department, the detectives continued to examine the floors and walls of the garage at several levels. On the cement floor of the seventh level, they soon found a set of car keys on a white holder, covered with a moist red substance. A short distance away from the keys, police also discovered a man's white handkerchief with moist reddish, blood-like stains and what appeared to be a dried red, paintlike substance.

Evidence technicians and detectives began collecting the reddish, bloodlike substances they were finding in and on the Buick on the eighth level that also created a trail leading down to the fifth level. These came from the stairwell leading from level 6A to 7A and from as low as the landing on level 5B. More scrapings and tape liftings were taken from the stairwell landing on level 7B. Inside the Electra, police also found and scraped more bloodlike substances from the car's gas pedal

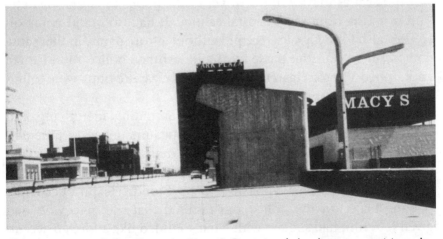

Crime scene at the Temple Street Garage (also known as Macy's parking lot) in New Haven.

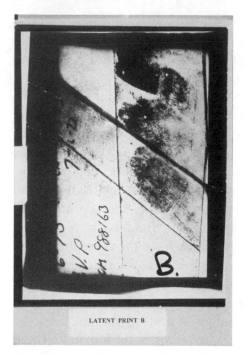

LATENT PRINT B

The latent prints found on this tissue box match the suspect's fingerprints.

and the carpeting and floor-board immediately around that area. Police also found reddish stains on the railing in the stairway leading from level nine to level ten. These were likewise scraped and collected. On the tenth level, police found a reddish substance on the Jeep parked there, which belonged to the New Haven Parking Authority, and these samples were also scraped and preserved.

Detectives soon began dusting the Buick for fingerprints. Several partial prints were discovered on the tissue box taken from the rear floor, immediately behind the driver's seat. Latent prints were lifted from the car's interior and its front-seat ashtrays. On the driver's side, police took one cigarette butt from the front seat's central ashtray. It had no brand name on it. They also found a sales receipt, without a store name, in that same compartment. On the passenger's-side ashtray, police found three cork-tipped Viceroy cigarette butts. Other cigarette butts were found in the car's rear ashtray.

While evidence technicians focused on finding, identifying, and collecting physical evidence, other investigators talked to potential witnesses and garage employees. The man who worked in the garage's ticket booth remembered receiving a parking ticket that had been moist with what appeared to be blood. He produced this parking ticket for the police and recalled that the man who had given it to him had spoken with what sounded like a foreign accent. After he had left the garage, this man had driven his car erratically through the garage's Frontage Street exit, going over the sidewalk as he left. The ticket taker was able to remember only the letters "AR" from the auto's license plates. He had no details to provide on the year, make, or model of this dark sedan. This witness was able to describe the driver as a Caucasian having long, dark hair and a thin build. He was a young man but not a kid.

Police talked to other eyewitnesses. They soon found another garage employee who said that he had seen a young woman running through levels five and six from a thin white male with longish black hair who appeared to be in his later twenties. The female, he remembered, wore no shoes. The Temple Street Garage was designed to fold into the heart of New Haven's central business district and Malley's department store. Bill Swanson,* a twenty-year-old employee at the store, was on his lunch break at the time of the murder, and he, along with two female store employees, had entered the garage to smoke marijuana on that July midday. Swanson told police that he'd seen a dark-haired younger man, with a moustache, chasing a young woman through the eighth level. In his initial statements, he omitted telling the investigators that he was stoned when he'd made his observations.

By 4:30 that afternoon, the identified body of Penney Serra had been moved the half mile or so to Yale–New Haven Hospital. Dr. David Papermaster, chief pathologist at the hospital, had phoned Dr. Elliot Gross, at that time Connecticut's chief medical examiner, and had been given approval for conducting an immediate autopsy of the victim's remains. A police photographer was present and took photos with a Polaroid and a black-and-white camera. Penney Serra had been wearing a plain, blue knit dress, with the brand name Eedra. Under this garment was a white half-slip that had a crotch, with the brand name Velrose. The victim had worn a purple bra, brand name Warner, and white, flowered underpants, size 7. Faint traces of semen were later found in both the half-slip and the underpants, though not enough to provide any serological typing, and it was unclear if these garments had been subjected to a thorough washing since the semen had been deposited. Penney Serra had also worn two gold chain necklaces, one with an Italian horn pendant.

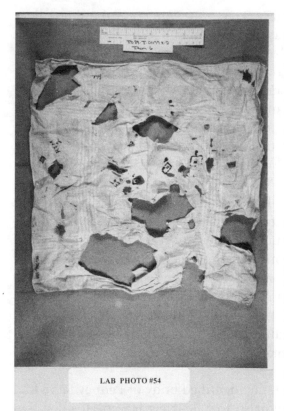

LAB PHOTO #54

A white handkerchief was found on the garage floor next to the victim's car. Samples have been removed from the handkerchief by cutting.

There was an observable scrape wound on the victim's right wrist, possibly by an assailant's hand. There were similar scrape wounds on her left knee and on her inner left ankle. There was what appeared to be a knife wound to her right little finger at the first joint, plus a cut alongside her right eye. Early in the autopsy, Dr. Papermaster found an abrasion to the right temporal region of the head, and he determined that this had occurred immediately prior to the victim's death. This wound was not visible without the use of a magnifying glass, and there was no means for determining if it was the result of a blow or a fall. There was no fracture of the skull. Dr. Papermaster then examined the victim's chest cavity. This area was completely full of blood. There was an entry wound, caused by a thin, sharp instrument, between the fifth and sixth ribs that penetrated the right ventricle of the heart. Dr. Papermaster told the police detectives that the weapon that had caused this fatal wound had a maximum width of one and one-eighth inches. Its minimum length, based on his probe of the weapon's path, was three inches. This stab wound resulted in intense internal bleeding and was the cause of death. Dr. Papermaster said that it was impossible to determine if the murder weapon was a knife, but that this object had to have been made of strong material, and that the fatal thrust did not bring with it any "sawing" effect. He also could not say definitively if the weapon had a serrated edge, though he could find no evidence of this type of blade design.

Police quickly established that Penney Serra had been seeing Philip DeLieto, so Penney's former fiancé became a prime suspect. Detectives soon had a warrant to search DeLieto's home in nearby East Haven where they found a pair of scissors with one blade broken and with a reddish-brown stain that later tested positive as human blood. DeLieto proved cooperative and agreed to be interviewed by detectives later that day at police headquarters. Still unaware that Bill Swanson was under the influence of marijuana smoked that midday, police arranged a lineup at headquarters that would include DeLieto. However, on bringing Swanson into headquarters that evening, the witness happened to enter a hallway just as DeLieto was being moved to the viewing room. The two men jostled one another and exchanged glances. Swanson then went on to identify DeLieto as the man he had seen running after Penney Serra through the garage. Working with the department's sketch artist, Swanson created a drawing of a man, wearing a moustache, who closely resembled DeLieto. The two garage employee witnesses, including the man who took the bloodied parking ticket, also helped to make their own sketches that evening, but neither of them placed a moustache on his suspect's face, and neither rendering resembled DeLieto that closely.

The news of Penney Serra's murder caused shock and outrage in the local community. Connecticut's newspapers and television stations broadcast the terrible news and the stories about how the twenty-one-year-old had been stabbed to death in a public garage in broad daylight. Very quickly, Philip DeLieto emerged as the prime suspect, and the similarity of his name to that of his distant cousin, the chief of police, hit home with the average citizen. Police investigators were establishing that DeLieto's relationship with Penney Serra seemed to be on shaky ground, a fact that only further fueled

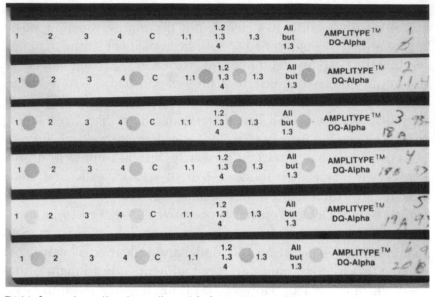

DNA found on the handkerchief matched the suspect's DNA profile. The figure shows DQA1–DNA typing result.

police and public suspicion toward him. But detectives also began to bear down hard on DeLieto's alibi, that he had worked that entire lunchtime at his family's downtown restaurant. Members of DeLieto's immediate family swore he had been working side by side with them during the timespan when the murder occurred. Many customers also corroborated DeLieto's story. One such customer was a navy commander who ran the recruiting station located near the luncheonette, and he remembered seeing DeLieto over the entire lunch hour. Years later, this individual would amend his statement, claiming that there had been a twenty-minute gap in that timeframe in which he did not see the suspect. Since the luncheonette was a mile or so away from the garage in busy noontime traffic, even this one change did not shake DeLieto's airtight alibi.

The New Haven community did not seem to want to hear about an alibi for Philip DeLieto. There is that subtle fault line between healthy skepticism and very unhealthy cynicism. The skeptic is rightly concerned about something going wrong, while the cynic sits back and seems to enjoy it when things go sour. Largely because of Ben DiLieto's being the New Haven police chief, many people continued to cling to the idea that Philip DeLieto was being ignored as a suspect and was able to get away with murder because the chief had ordered a cover-up. I came to know Ben DiLieto well and can vouch for his excellent character. He was not the type of person to meddle with any kind of a departmental investigation, let alone such a heinous and brutal murder. Ironically, it was Nicholas Pastore who ran the police investigation, and he was not close to Ben DiLieto. In later years, the two openly clashed over other matters. Yet Pastore, to his credit, vowed that Chief DiLieto absolutely did not interfere in the way this case was investigated.

Excluding Philip DeLieto as their man, the police ran into a stone wall. Who would do such a horrible thing to a good-natured, young, and pretty woman, all in broad daylight and in a public place, where the chances of being caught were extremely high? The police noted that no money was taken from Penney Serra's wallet, and the killer had left two gold chains around her neck. There seemed to be no effort to steal the Buick Electra, though it was probable that the murderer had driven the car in the garage, from the upper floor, down to the eighth level. There were no ripped articles of clothing or other evidence of a sexual assault. There were only a few possible motives that would drive someone—in all probability the man witnesses saw running after Penney Serra that day—to commit such a crime. Did he know her, and was this a crime of passion? With the limited amount of forensic evidence and the technology of that time, police did not seem to have very many directions in which to take their investigation.

Four additional, experienced detectives were assigned to work with Detective Pastore full-time on the Penney Serra murder. This was, in part, a public gesture to mollify the early critics who were demanding a quick solution to this notorious crime, especially in light of the Philip DeLieto dead end. Detective Pastore also announced that, since a mechanic's rag had been found on the floor in the back of the Serra car, his investigators were going to interview owners and managers of all the gas stations and auto repair shops in

New Haven County. At that time, a rough estimate put the total of these stations and shops at twenty-five hundred. This seemed like an extremely daunting task, but one well worth the effort if police could find the person who had been in downtown New Haven that noon. Let's do the arithmetic on just how daunting a task this really was. With four detectives calling on five auto shops a day, one hundred stations could be covered in a week, still leaving several hours apiece for each of them to follow other leads and perform other duties. The entire canvassing could have been completed in twenty-five weeks. The police did undertake this tedious task. But these investigators did not travel out to Waterbury, which is New Haven County's second-largest city. As facts would prove many years later, this was a very regrettable oversight.

In October of 1973, police received blood-typing results from the Toxicology Laboratory at the Hartford Health Department. Bloodstains found on the tenth-level stairwell were type A, which was Penney Serra's blood type. The suspect's was found to be type O. These are both very common blood types. There were several identifiable latent fingerprints found in the car by the New Haven police's ID unit. These fingerprints were compared with the known fingerprints of Penney Serra and the members of her family. Most of the fingerprints were identified, except for the bloody fingerprints on the tissue box in the backseat area of the car. These fingerprints were not identifiable and did not originate with the victim or any member of her family. The fingerprints also did not originate with Philip DeLieto. Subsequently, the unidentifiable fingerprints were sent to the Connecticut State Police Identification Unit to search against a state fingerprint databank, a complicated manual, ten-point class system in use at that time. To manually search a million fingerprint cards, properly filed, would take a qualified technician a total of fifty-two years. This was, effectively, an impossible job. These fingerprints were also sent to the FBI's fingerprint-identification division, but no identification was made. The New Haven police continued to look for witnesses, while John Serra, the victim's loving father, slowly began to start his own campaign to find Penney's killer. However, with the notable exception of New Haven's two

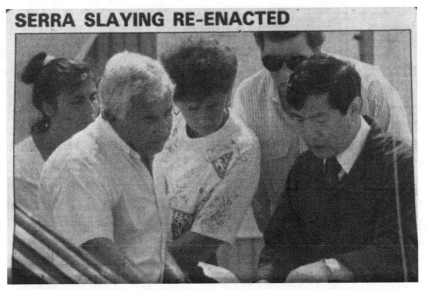

SERRA SLAYING RE-ENACTED

Dr. Lee meets Mr. John Serra, father of the victim, and family members at the Temple Street Garage to reinvestigate the case.

daily newspapers, both owned by the *New Haven Register,* the media began moving on to other stories. The first anniversary of Penney's death came and went, and her murder began to appear unsolvable, one of the classic characteristics of the cold case. As Mr. Serra began to suggest in his advertising campaign, his daughter's killer was at large in the New Haven area, an assumption made by Penney's distraught father that would someday prove eerily prophetic.

As I said earlier in this chapter, I only arrived in America in 1965, and I would not move to the New Haven area until ten years later. In supporting my family and meeting the demands of a full course schedule, I was quite challenged at this time. I also had the task of mastering English, a language that was completely foreign to me. My life was completely filled with numerous duties and obligations that I was only too happy to undertake. I did not have the time or the inclination to follow closely any criminal investigations, not even the Martha Moxley murder in Greenwich, which occurred in October of my first year in Connecticut. Even in 1975, after I accepted an instructor's post at the University of New Haven, located in West Haven, I was far too busy with establishing course curricula and reading lists, which precluded my delving into a local case like the Penney Serra murder. Besides, Margaret and I had our two children to raise and educate. Work took up a good part of my day, but I believe very strongly in family bonds, and I wanted to spend as much time as possible with my mother, my wife, and my two children. I am now extremely proud of my family, and Margaret and I share great satisfaction in their personal and professional accomplishments.

I was not the only one moving to the New Haven area in the midseventies. In the summer of 1977, my coauthor, Tom O'Neil, moved his family to New Haven, where he would head up, for a time, a new regional magazine. In the fall of that year, Tom was busy working in downtown New Haven, at the principal state courthouse, when he lost track of the time and found that his car had been towed to the Serra family's auto garage. When he arrived to claim his auto and pay the thirty-five-dollar fine, John Serra greeted Tom and asked him if he recognized the Serra name. When Tom's reply was no, John Serra quickly filled him in on the details of his daughter's murder and the fact that the case had not yet been solved. I relate this anecdote to underscore the degree to which Penney Serra's father was preoccupied by the death of his daughter and his desire to catch her murderer. The phrase *thirst for justice* seems very apt to me. Mr. Serra's grief and his outrage over Penney's killer still being at large and free must have made him feel like a man in the desert, wanting to quench his terrible thirst with a cool glass of water. John Serra is not the only individual I have come to know who had this deep drive to bring to justice someone who had cruelly taken the life of a child, a wife, or some other loved one. This palpable grief by John Serra, which was so strong that it could be termed his obsession, is what helped bring this case to a successful conclusion. Similarly, Dorthy Moxley's purposeful campaign to see her daughter's killer finally brought to justice (as discussed later) provides another constructive example of how effectively a grieving parent can help drive a long and ultimately successful murder investigation.

The Serra case did not turn cold due to any lack of interest by the

New Haven Police Department. The local media, particularly the *New Haven Register*, continued to cover the case and, at anniversaries of the crime, to review all of the evidence. Sadly enough, the community didn't seem able to shake the notion that, somehow and in some way, Philip DeLieto had been spared because his distant relative served as chief of police. This suspicion persisted despite there being many nonfamily witnesses available who provided Penney Serra's outgoing boyfriend with an airtight alibi. Since nature abhors a vacuum, there weren't, for more than a decade, many other avenues for the media to explore. The suspicion still directed at Mr. DeLieto must have made his life very uncomfortable.

Things changed in 1984. Anthony Golino had been a star pitcher on the Wilbur Cross High School baseball teams in the late sixties and, as it developed, knew Penney Serra. Golino and his wife, Melanie,* had dated throughout the later sixties and were finally married in 1977. The couple had a very stormy relationship, and, in 1982, after the birth of a son, the two separated and then divorced. At the time of their breakup, Melanie Golino went to the police and told them that Anthony had beat her and, on several occasions, threatened to kill her, essentially saying, "I will do to you, what I did to Penney Serra."[4] There had also been reports that Golino had dated Penney Serra when police initially became interested in him in the midseventies. But Melanie Golino's allegations now brought Anthony Golino into the small circle of suspects in this investigation. Consequently, Golino was called into police headquarters and was extensively questioned about those potentially incriminating statements, which the suspect denied having made. Golino, police noted, also had a one-inch scar on his left hand, one that he was unable to explain.

In the New Haven community, Golino had enjoyed a good reputation and had, for years, been the coach of a successful American Legion baseball team. When questioned, Golino told police that he believed that his blood was type O, which was the same as Penney Serra's assailant. However, the police did not test Golino's blood at that time. Detectives also pursued eyewitness accounts that arose reporting Golino and Penney had been seeing one another in the summer of 1973. One witness said she remembered seeing the two talking over drinks at a local club, and another recalled the two of them having a spat on a street corner.

In the summer of 1984, the New Haven police applied for and were granted an arrest warrant charging Anthony Golino with the murder of Penney Serra. By now, Golino had been divorced from Melanie for two years. Many in the New Haven area were unconvinced of his guilt and were suspicious that Golino was a sacrificial lamb whom police had found to stand in for Philip DeLieto, whose distant cousin, former police chief Ben DiLieto, had been elected the mayor of New Haven. Golino's fortunes improved dramatically, though, when he was able, through the public defender's office, to retain Hugh Keefe as his defense counsel. I have known Hugh Keefe since shortly after I joined the University of New Haven in 1975 to develop a forensic science program. I consider him one of the best defense lawyers I have ever known. Handsome and redheaded and armed with a sharp Irish wit, Hugh Keefe is known far and wide as a prodigious worker and a charismatic litigator. Golino's defense was going to be in excellent hands. Mary Galvin, the assistant to State's Attorney Arnold Markle, who prosecuted the Golino case, is also an old and dear friend of mine and an individual who is widely respected as a superb attorney and an excellent teacher. I initially was introduced to Mary Galvin by Arnold Markle, one of the most legendary prosecutors in Connecticut history. Even today, Mary and I often give lectures and teach together at attorney, police, and arson investigator conferences and training workshops.

Though Golino was arrested in 1984, the prosecution was not ready for trial until the middle of 1987. This delay was due in large part to defense motions put forward by Keefe, one of which centered on the five-year statute of limitations for murder in effect in 1973. Others hammered at the prosecution's lack of any direct evidence linking Anthony Golino to the crime scene or providing a motive for Golino to kill Penney Serra. Instead of being thin and short, like the man witnesses described chasing Penney Serra through the Temple Street Garage, Golino was husky and taller. Keefe also called into sharp question the authenticity of Melanie Golino's claims that her former husband had threatened her with death while invoking Penney Serra's name. Finally, in August of 1987, on the eve of the trial's opening, Mary Galvin executed a search warrant for Golino's blood, which she sent to my laboratory to be tested. Rather than his blood being type O, the results showed that Anthony Golino had type A blood, similar to the victim's blood. Hugh Keefe quickly asked for and was granted a dismissal of the murder charges against Golino. Thus, another time-consuming chapter in the long history of this case was closed. The price of this charge for Golino was still very high. Within sixteen days of his being cleared of the murder, his father suffered a fatal heart attack. His mother died within the next six months. He became estranged from his brother and sister. Throughout the ordeal, Golino lost sixty pounds. Golino later sued for false arrest, but in 1993 a federal judge denied his claims.[5] The former baseball star and diligent coach had his name very badly tarnished and was never able to get his life back on track. To this day, Anthony Golino remains one of the victims of this crime.

During the eighties, the New Haven police also pursued another prime suspect, Martin Cooratal. His dental bill was found on the dashboard of the Serra family's Buick Electra. He was Albanian by birth and worked at a luncheon restaurant on Chapel Street, a few doors down from where Penney Serra had worked. The eyewitness in the Temple Street Garage's booth, who had taken the blood-stained parking ticket shortly after 1:00 PM on July 16, had reported that the driver had spoken to him in what seemed like a foreign accent. Also, Cooratal had relatively long, dark hair, was thin, and otherwise resembled witnesses' descriptions of the man who chased Penney Serra through the parking garage. Police, from the first, had called Cooratal in for questioning, but, like Philip DeLieto, detectives had encountered witnesses who placed him at his workstation in the luncheonette. After their unsuccessful prosecution of Golino, the police refocused their attention on Cooratal, who had moved away from the New Haven area to Texas. Over the decades, New Haven detectives attempted on two occasions to obtain arrest warrants for Cooratal, charging him with Penney Serra's murder, and both of these were refused by the courts for lack of evidence.

Because this case was not going anywhere, and due, in large part, to John Serra's very public questions about how his daughter's murder was being handled, pressure built for a wider investigation. In early 1987, Arnold Markle, the outstanding state's attorney for New Haven and a close personal friend of mine, initiated a review of the Serra murder. But, unfortunately, Markle passed away in December of 1987. That same month, John Kelly, the chief state's attorney for Connecticut, stepped in to investigate the case. Jack Kelly is an extremely hardworking, very intelligent, and highly competent attorney. He and his wife, Dr. Freida Kelly, became good friends of Margaret and me. We have participated in several lecture trips to Taiwan and China. He had the Serra case jointly reassigned to the Connecticut State Police Forensic Science Laboratory, which I headed, and the State's Attorney's Office of New Haven, now headed by Michael Dearington, a very handsome and very capable prosecutor. This move rankled members of the New Haven Police Department who had worked for years to solve the Serra murder. Despite this, together both offices moved forward as a new task force. After reviewing all of the case's witness statements and investigative reports, we were able to establish a timeline for the death of Penney Serra. However, we saw that there were some inconsistencies within the witnesses' statements and the actual timeline analysis. After several meetings with the chief state's attorney, Jack Kelly, and the New Haven state's attorney, Mike Dearington, we made the decision to go back to the original crime scene, the parking garage, to conduct a crime scene reconstruction.

The decision also caused a sensation in the local and state media. The CBS newsmagazine Sunday evening show *60 Minutes* even sent their star reporter, Mike Wallace, to New Haven to review the Serra murder. Then, in February of 1988, in a twenty-minute segment seen by an estimated twenty million Americans, Wallace and his CBS producers focused national attention on Philip DeLieto, Penney Serra's boyfriend and former fiancé. Television, by its very nature, excites people more than the print media or radio. Once the *60 Minutes* segment aired, it landed like a bombshell. As I've noted, a lingering sense of doubt persisted among many because of Phil

DeLieto's distant relationship to the former chief of police, and his identification in a police lineup focused more attention on Phil DeLieto. This was despite the eyewitness being a twenty-year-old who was high on marijuana (as later revealed) when he'd observed the killer chasing his victim through the garage, and not to mention the fact that the witness, Bill Swanson, had actually jostled Phil DeLieto, making eye contact, at police headquarters shortly before he'd made his identification. And all of this was on top of the fact that Swanson was the only one of the three eyewitnesses who'd said that the assailant wore a moustache, as Philip DeLieto did.

In retrospect, the *60 Minutes* airing of the Serra case proved beneficial, since this TV show intensified and widened public interest in the case. Yet I cannot help feeling sadness for both Philip and my friend, the late chief Ben DiLieto. The Monday morning after the segment aired, Ben DiLieto told reporters that he had never, in all his years of public service, been so "disappointed" by an event as he was by the show's implying that he helped cover up Philip DeLieto's role in the Serra murder. Ben DiLieto was getting ready to retire from public life, and the storm caused by this production came at a very bad time. Also, Philip DiLieto had married and was quietly going about his own business when this bombshell landed. Mayor DiLieto carried through with his long-standing plans not to run for reelection the next year. He continued to appear as the honored speaker at a number of civic dinners and testimonials. The community, which had grown used to the charges aired by CBS, now tended to discount any meddling by him in the Serra case. With his decades of successful public service, Ben DiLieto had won the public's trust, and CBS now seemed to be viewed as an outside agitator. I remember Ben appearing at dinners in the nineties, when he would have to leave the dais to indulge his habit of chain-smoking, as many police officers do. This chain-smoking probably was a contributing factor to Ben's early death in 1996.

Once we had become directly involved in the Serra case, our staff in the State Police Forensic Science Laboratory went to work to reexamine all of the physical evidence that had been gathered in order to use the scientific evidence to verify or disprove every witness's statement. On Sunday, September 10, 1989, we pulled together members of our staff, state police investigators, a key detective from the New Haven police, and prosecutors, who all assembled at the Temple Street Garage. There, we created a crime reenactment, one that provided, as nearly as possible, the times of the various components of the murder of Penney Serra. Those present with me included Jack Kelly, chief state's attorney; Michael Dearington, New Haven state's attorney; Kenneth Zercie and Dr. Jack Hubball, lead criminalists in our office, and their associate, Bob O'Brien, a bright, young forensic star; William Paetzold, a criminalist trainee from our office; Capt. Donald Beausejour from the New Haven Police Department; and other inspectors from both the chief state's attorney's office and the New Haven state's attorney's office.

This crime scene reenactment consisted of two major considerations: a precise reestablishment of the crime scenes and the setting out in detail the sequence of events that occurred in the midday of July 16, 1973. This was accomplished through use of the documents, photos, diagrams, and measurements recorded on that date by the New Haven Police Department. The location of each piece of physical evidence and when it was found were reestablished. Numbered markers were utilized to represent bloodstains, tiremarks, and other relevant evidence, all placed in their appropriate locations. We then reviewed the witnesses' statements: to verify the continuity of the events described by the various witnesses and to verify their positions and viewpoints on July 16, 1973. After that we performed a reconstruction of the vehicular activity prior to and immediately after the murder. We were able to achieve this through both witness statements and the times recorded on the two garage parking tickets. Since the original location of the assailant's vehicle was unknown, we were able to establish only a likely timeframe for when the suspect left the victim's vehicle on level eight.

Later that month, we compiled the information and the evidence into a series of case facts:

- The Temple Street Garage was the primary crime scene. The incident more likely started on the seventh floor and continued to the tenth-floor staircase.

- Using the original crime scene photographs, we saw that the blood trail through the garage came from the left side of an injured person. This coincided with the fact that the latent thumbprint found on the tissue box on the floor behind the driver's seat in the victim's Buick was most likely from the assailant's left thumb.
- Penney Serra died from a single stab wound, administered by a single-sided, knifelike object measuring approximately three-quarters of an inch in length by one-quarter inch wide, to her heart.
- Penney Serra's death fell into one of two categories: the victim and the suspect were well acquainted and their meeting was prearranged or the victim and the suspect were total strangers and the killing was an act of totally random chance, perhaps the action of a psychotic.
- The bloodstain and blood patterns found on the tenth-floor stairwell indicate that the victim had reached at least the third step. Subsequently, her wound contacted the third step, causing a flowing and contact-type transfer blood smear pattern. The victim's body then had fallen in a downward direction toward the landing of the stairwell to its final, fetal-like position.
- Based on the crime scene patterns, rape and robbery did not appear to be motives for this assault and the victim's death. The traces of sperm found, one apiece, on the victim's underpants and on her legged half-slip, both in the crotch area, were not mixed with any vaginal fluid. This meant that, in all probability, the sperm had been ejaculated outside the undergarments, the date of this deposit being impossible to determine.
- The origin of the semen DNA was never established. Whether the semen stains had been consumed by earlier investigation or due to the garments' being put through a light washing could not be determined.

Our report also focused on the bloodstain evidence in and on the Serra family Buick. Since all of this blood was from a human source whose blood type was O, this fact suggested that this was the assailant's blood. The blood evidence also appeared as a trail along the garage's levels five, six, seven, and eight. The blood droplets came from a vertical source, meaning that the assailant was moving while he bled from his left side, probably from his left hand. Penney Serra's blood evidence, found only on the stairwell on the tenth level, was type A. These facts suggested that the victim had struggled with her assailant where her car was parked on the ninth level, and she had been responsible for the substantial cut inflicted on the assailant's left hand. The attacker had then pursued his victim through the ninth level to the tenth level of the garage. Two witnesses had given statements that they'd seen a thin, Caucasian man, carrying a shiny object, chasing a young woman. Running for her life, Penney Serra dashed up a stairwell to the tenth level, where she found herself trapped at the foot of the blind stairwell. There she was then stabbed one time, a wound that extended into her heart, causing her to die in a timespan of ninety seconds or so.

According to the two witnesses in the garage, Penney Serra's attacker returned to the ninth level after a few seconds. He then ran to the Buick, where he found the victim's keys and started her car. He then drove the car erratically from the ninth level back down to the garage's eighth level, where he parked the victim's car at an extreme angle, where it was found. Bill Swanson, the Malley's employee who was under the influence of marijuana, also saw a man driving the blue Buick. The killer, leaving a blood trail, then ran to the seventh level, where it is highly probable he had parked his own car, got into it, and erratically drove out of the garage onto Frontage Street, after paying and handing in the blood-smeared parking ticket. Based on the time stamped onto this ticket, the assailant left the crime scene at 1:01 PM. While getting into his own vehicle on the seventh level, the suspect dropped the blood-smeared keys and the white handkerchief on the garage floor.

Our report covered each piece of physical evidence. One was the brownish wig found by the garage employee on the railing of the stairwell leading from the tenth to the ninth levels. Under the microscope, all of the hairs of the wig were consistent with one another, except for two hair fragments, which had the characteristics of Afro-American hair. Before being bagged, the wig had been moved from place to place in the garage by investigators and witnesses the afternoon of the murder, and, hence, these two hair fragments could have been picked up during these multiple contacts. Thus, there was never any forensic significance attached to the wig. However, there was an enormous amount of significance placed on the four sets of unexplainable latent fingerprints found either in or on the Serra car or on objects found inside the Buick. By *latent fingerprints*, I refer to fingerprints that are not visible to the naked eye and must be treated with physical or chemical methods to become visible. Three of these prints were completely unidentifiable, and the fourth, from the bloodied parking ticket, was only a bloody print.

Not until late 1990 did computer imaging become a reality. These latent print images were digitized into a computer and visualized on a high-resolution monitor, then were passed through filters and gray-scaling programs to produce the best possible images. At my direction, laboratory scientists at the University of Connecticut conducted an exhaustive, computerized reexamination of these prints, a process that included photographic reproductions. Later, these latent images were sent to the Automated Fingerprint Identification System (AFIS), where file searches were made by many police agencies. These included the Metro Dade County (Miami) Police Department, the Baltimore Police Department, the California Department of Justice, the Royal Canadian Mounted Police, and, of course, the FBI. No identifications were reported, however. All the cooperating agencies indicated that they would regularly search their compatible fingerprint files, and, should an individualizing match be found, they would promptly notify us. This type of cooperation and commitment to justice warmed my heart.

On Sunday, September 24, 1989, two weeks after we conducted the reenactment of the crime at the Temple Street Garage, the *New Haven Register* published an extensive review of the Serra case, complete with a rendering showing the murderer's route through the parking garage.[6] During an interview for this story with the *Register*'s Nick Povinelli, I said that advances in latent-fingerprint and DNA technology were improving dramatically. Thus, I predicted, I could hold out hope that someday this case could be solved and the murderer of Penney Serra would be brought to justice. Several prominent New Haven defense lawyers expressed their skepticism over this case ever being successfully prosecuted, citing the time span since the murder had been committed as was well as the unsuccessful prosecution of previous suspects as critical factors. As though sensing the major break that half a decade later would help break this case, Ira Grudberg, a famous and brilliant attorney, did say that "minus something totally unforeseen, it's [the Serra murder] probably something that can't be proved."

Reporter Nick Povinelli's in-depth review also spotlighted the determination of John Serra, Penney's father, who had fought for sixteen-plus years for justice for his beloved daughter. According to the story, Mr. Serra had even recently posted a sign on his Forbes Avenue business that said, "Use Caution in the Temple Street Garage." He continued to run his monthly ads calling for justice in the *New Haven Register*. John Serra also told Povinelli: "This is not an obsession with me. It's that . . . I'm determined . . . I don't live it twenty-four hours a day. I just try to think twenty-four hours a day . . . that's all." He added that he felt he was doing what any other father of a murdered daughter would do. Mr. Serra concluded with a review of the renewed investigative efforts by the state's attorney's office and the state police forensic science laboratory: "I believe they put a lot of time and effort into it. I'm hoping for the best. But I'll deal with that when the time comes."[7] The Sunday *New Haven Register* had a circulation of more than one hundred thousand at that time and a pass-along readership well above that figure. Thousands of copies of the paper were sold in the Waterbury area, and one has to wonder if a man whose fingerprints were now in AFIS databanks would read John Serra's comments in that news story and would fear being apprehended.

Another five years went by, with more work and more frustration. John Serra remained his tenacious self, yet he never showed my staff or me anything but his respect. He occasionally called me on the phone to check on the case's progress. He also visited me in my office a couple of times, to hear me, in person, explain the procedures we were employing as well as the case's progress. We all identified with his feelings, and I deeply admired his fighting spirit, battling for justice for his daughter, who had now been dead for more than two decades. Rosemary Serra, John's younger daughter, had long since grown up and matured into a loving and capable lady. Those of us who regularly revisited the evidence and studied the facts of this case hoped we might suddenly unearth some tiny clue somewhere that would lead us to the suspect who committed this terrible murder. Deep in my heart, there were times when I wondered if the day of reckoning would ever dawn. Like the other professionals, I simply had to go on this long route of pursuing any and all possibilities while I went about my other duties and responsibilities. We all hoped that all of our hard work and painstaking investigation would pay off.

In 1994 something did happen. I know that critics of human behavior say that people never really change, that individuals cannot break away from bad habits and behavior patterns, no matter their best intentions or their religious devotion. The newer Megan's Law reflects this philosophy, in a limited way. According to national studies, the recidivism rate of sex crimes is disproportionately high. Once a person has committed a sexual crime, particularly against a child, there is a strong possibility that the offender, even after he has served his sentence, will very likely repeat that type of crime. In the summer of 1994, Edward R. Grant of Waterbury beat his then-fiancée so fiercely that she was hospitalized. This victim reported Grant's assault to the local police, and he was arrested. Subsequently, Edward Grant was fingerprinted. Grant was then fifty-one and had worked most of his adult life at his family's auto repair and towing business in Waterbury. In 1971, already married, Grant had been a member of the Connecticut National Guard and, while on his six months of active duty in South Carolina during the Vietnam War, had been injured in a Jeep accident. Depending on who is telling the tale, the intoxicated Grant was driving the Jeep or was simply a passenger when the vehicle rolled over. The injuries that Grant sustained resulted in a steel plate being placed in his head, and he was given an administrative discharge from the service. Grant returned to his home in Waterbury and went back to work for his family's successful business. The long-term effects of his injury were that he suffered from memory loss and severe mood swings.

In the later seventies, Grant and his first wife divorced. They had two children, a boy and a girl. Quiet by nature, Grant remained close to his family and regularly visited his children. Grant's niece later would say that her uncle was violent by nature and his outbursts frightened her. This young woman could not have been too surprised when Edward Grant was arrested in 1994 for badly beating his fiancée, though those charges were later dropped. There was a far graver consequence to this alleged assault for Grant, though. His complete set of fingerprints was now automatically filed in the state AFIS system. In 1997 a Connecticut/Rhode Island fingerprint database scored a hit on Edward Grant's left thumbprint: it matched the bloody partial print on the tissue box that lay on the floor behind the driver's seat of the car driven by Penney Serra on July 16, 1973.

The identification of this print electrified those of us who had been waiting for years to catch a break in this case. Edward Grant's age, occupation, and track record for violence with women further galvanized investigators. Working methodically, investigators called on Grant and advised him of the fingerprint match, being careful first to provide him with his *Miranda* rights. When Grant could not account for his print being at the crime scene, police offered him what they termed as a way for him to exonerate himself: investigators asked for a sample of his blood. Grant, who had not consulted an attorney at this point, refused. In and of itself, this further intrigued the investigative team. Investigators then applied for and were granted a warrant to draw samples of Edward Grant's blood. This was then sent to our laboratory for DNA analysis. The DNA evidence came back and indicated that there was at least a 300-million-to-1 chance that the type O blood found at the Serra crime scene was Edward Grant's. Still working methodically, detectives arrested Edward Grant in June of 1999 for the murder of Penney Serra. Grant's bail was set at $1 million, which, with the help of his extended family, he was able to post. Sitting in the backseat of a police cruiser after he was initially arrested, Grant commented to an officer next to him that the recent arrest of a railroad serial killer in Texas had come "from a single thumbprint, too."

Sadly enough, John Serra had already died in November of 1998. This was eight months prior to Edward Grant's being arrested and formally charged with the Penney Serra murder. Investigators, however, had informed Mr. Serra about the match of Grant's thumbprint and the gathering DNA evidence that further incriminated this suspect. However, John Serra never lived to see justice in his daughter's murder ultimately served. His surviving daughter, Penney's younger sister, Rosemary, was alive and living in the area, the sole survivor of her original family of four. And somewhere, after Grant's arrest, Philip DeLieto had to be quietly applauding. Characteristically enough, Anthony Golino declaimed Grant's arrest, asserting that this defendant was also innocent and that the murder would never be solved. Though Penney Serra had been a humble and quiet young lady, she still had many friends and supporters in the area who shared in the jubilation over the arrest of Grant. This excitement was felt, I'm sure, by the thousands of others who had followed this case since its inception. Those of us who had worked directly on the investigation did not even have time to enjoy this excitement. That's because there are thousands of other cases waiting for us yet to solve by finding that one clue. And we all knew in our hearts that there was a long legal battle still to be fought to see this murderer brought to justice.

THE SERRA TRIAL

Thomas J. Ullmann headed the New Haven Public Defender's Office. At the time, he was a thoroughly respected defense counsel in his later forties, an individual whose graying and trimmed beard gave him an elfin look. Many years ago I met him for the first time. Since then, we on the prosecution side of the courtroom continue to respect him for his dedication to duty, for his ability to attract bright and conscientious lawyers to his staff, and for his devotion to excellent research on each and every case. In the summer of 1999, Edward Grant did not have the money needed to retain private defense counsel, so the Serra murder charges were referred to the public defender's office and ultimately to Tom Ullmann, who would lead the defense team. Given the fact that Ullmann was personally heading the defense, Edward Grant, in my estimation, had caught a very lucky break.

Under Ullmann, the defense team immediately challenged Grant's prosecution on the grounds that the charge specifically violated the five-year statute of limitations for murder in effect in 1973, and the legal ethics of trying a case that was more than twenty-five years old. Ullmann also attacked the forensic evidence in the case, claiming that the storage provided at the Connecticut state laboratories in both Hartford and Meriden were inadequate to the task of properly preserving the blood and fingerprint evidence. The white handkerchief found on the seventh level of the parking garage, with its blood and paint smears, was singled out by the defense as having been corrupted to the point that it was unsuitable for any further scientific testing. The defense team argued in a series of motions that during the hot summers the blood samples had decayed. Ideally, Grant's lawyers argued, this human blood residue should have been stored in facilities with refrigeration instead of in storerooms where the thermometer at times climbed into the nineties. Also, the handkerchief had been handled by dozens of investigators and laboratory scientists over the years, some of whom cut swatches for testing purposes. Thus, the sheer volume of all of this treatment had corroded the evidence.

After twenty years of service, in 1998 I retired from my post as director of the Connecticut State Police Forensic Science Laboratory, only to become, at the personal request of Gov. John Rowland, the state's commissioner of the Department of Public Safety. This new task meant that I had many administrative responsibilities to tend to, such as the procurement and distribution of a state-of-the-art computer system to all State Police vehicles, which provided officers in the field with instant access to thousands of important files. Because of the hundreds of hours I had already invested in the Serra case, I took a close personal interest in preparing the scientific data needed to respond to the motions that Edward Grant's defense team had filed for a dismissal of the case on the grounds that the scientific evidence had become unusable.

The prosecution team worked hard to defeat these defense motions. Assistant State's Attorney James G. Clark was given the assignment to prosecute Edward Grant, and, from the outset, I thought that Michael Dearington, the New Haven chief state's attorney, had made an excellent choice. Jim Clark, also in his later forties, was a very competent and experienced attorney who already had several successful prosecutions to his credit. Clark and Tom Ullmann had served as adversaries in court on a number of occasions, so each knew his opponent well. Elaine Pagliaro was now assistant director of the state's forensic science laboratory. She had worked with me there for almost twenty years, and I was confident that our laboratory scientists could prove, beyond a reasonable doubt, that the blood, fingerprint, and other scientific evidence had been adequately preserved to the very best of our abilities. To do this, the state's forensic experts demonstrated that the evidence had been subjected to extremely tight chain-of-custody practices and had been correctly preserved to the best of our ability at that time. Elaine testified at the hearings conducted on the defense team's motions to dismiss. The prosecution cited long-established blood-evidence practices, accepted by courts in previous cases, as evidence that proper precautions and treatment had been taken. In the summer of 2001, the prosecution prevailed, and all of the defense motions to rule out the scientific evidence were rejected.

On Monday, April 29, 2002, veteran Superior Court judge Jon C. Blue gaveled to order the trial of Edward Grant, now fifty-nine, for the 1973 murder of Penney Serra.[8] Judge Blue, a mild and very competent judge, seemed an outstanding choice for the case, a jurist who was very familiar with scientific evidence and the prosecuting and defense teams. Judge Blue was well known for his pragmatic approach to running a trial, a jurist who had little patience for any petty sniping between opposing attorneys. He was also a judge who seemed particularly attentive to the difficult sacrifices and hardships jurors in longer trials endured and went out of his way to treat his jurors with deference. The selection of jurors for the Serra trial had

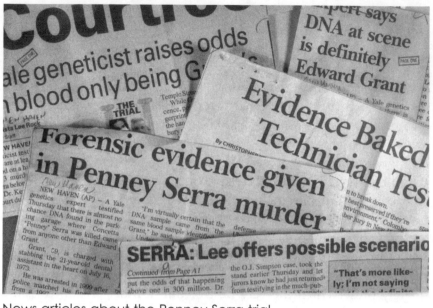

News articles about the Penney Serra trial.

been complicated by the years of publicity that the murder and its extended investigation had generated. During the voire dire hearings prior to the trial, both sides had to face the fact that a great many people in the New Haven metropolitan area knew something about the case. Therefore, under questioning, the prosecution and the defense were particularly alert for any prospective juror who had developed any kind of prejudgement on Edward Grant's guilt or innocence. Given our system of justice, a single juror could destroy the entire proceedings by his or her conduct, as one of the jury had done at the 1988 first trial of woodchipper murderer Richard Crafts. In that instance, one of the jurors had poisoned the jury's deliberations with his misconduct and finally walked out of the deliberations, precipitating a mistrial. Also, both sides at the Serra trial needed to probe juror prospects for any other latent problem, such as a close friendship with a member of the victim's family or some other personal factor that might come to light during the proceedings or after the trial ended.

Notwithstanding these problems, the jury-selection process

proceeded smoothly enough in this notorious case, and, within a week, a jury of six men and six women was seated. During his opening argument, defense counsel Thomas Ullmann argued that the New Haven Police Department had twice attempted, as recently as 1994, to arrest Martin Cooratal for the Serra murder and that there was more evidence to implicate him in the crime than there was against Edward Grant. Ullmann also went through the evidence originally brought by the police against Philip DeLieto. The defense was also planning to show jurors evidence that Edward Grant had been at his family's vacation cabin in Vermont on the date of the murder. They would say that Grant was detained there due to local flooding conditions caused by violent thunderstorms that summer. Prosecutor James Clark went directly to the blood and fingerprint evidence in his opening argument. He argued that both Cooratal and DeLieto were excluded as suspects since their DNA did not match the blood evidence found in the car or in the blood trails left by Penney Serra's attacker.

The prosecution team used two powerful examples of how modern criminal justice is able to provide complex information and data to those in the courtroom. At an estimated expense of $18,000, the prosecution had an architectural firm in Worcester, Massachusetts, create a detailed model of the Temple Street Garage, one made to an exact 1:48 scale. This ten-level, wooden mock-up measured eleven feet in length and provided jurors with a rendering of the garage so exact that each individual stair in the building was included. The model also provided prosecutors and their witnesses with a stage for displaying their theory of the crime, using different-colored, felt-tip pens to record their points.[9] They were able to demonstrate how Edward Grant had chased Penney Serra through the garage, trapped and fatally stabbed her in the tenth-level stairwell, and had finally driven her car to another level, where he jumped into his own vehicle and exited the garage. Jim Clark and others on his team merely had to point out locations and times to the jury to make the prosecution's points. The second visual aid that the prosecution used was a computer-controlled visual display system, which presented the scientific evidence on a big screen.

Blood spatter, DNA, and fingerprint testimony, correlated with photos, charts, and other slides, provided jurors with a visual display of the points we witnesses were explaining from the stand. These techniques, I feel, are very powerful, especially since the net effect tends to put a face on what jurors might otherwise find dry and highly technical information. I know that a number of defense lawyers object to this use of the computerized slides, but I am very confident that the courts will continue to permit the use of this technology, as long as the data presented are fair and accurate.

As the trial began its second week, the prosecution moved ahead to present its blood evidence and, specifically, the state's DNA testimony. Jim Clark called Elaine Pagliaro to the witness stand. She began by testifying to the relatively primitive nature of blood-analysis technology available in 1973, when forensic analysts could determine only whether a substance in question was human blood and, perhaps, from which of the four human blood types the sample came. She told the court that Penney's Serra's blood was type A and her assailant's was type O, the latter being found in and outside the Serra car, in a blood trail through the garage, and on a handkerchief left on the seventh level. Elaine was also laying the groundwork for the state's DNA experts.

But the proceedings in Judge Blue's sixth-floor courtroom were disrupted that day. Anthony Golino, who had been in attendance each day of the trial, suddenly became an issue. During a recess, Judge Blue was advised by one of his clerks that Golino had been overheard making derogatory and obscene comments about the testimony of one of the New Haven police detectives who had originally worked the case. The matter under discussion was Philip DeLieto's early cooperation with police and his having made physical contact with eyewitness Bill Swanson, who later selected DeLieto out of eight individuals in a lineup as the man he'd seen driving Penney Serra's Buick in the Temple Street Garage. Judge Blue sternly rebuked Golino for his conduct and threw him out of the courtroom for the rest of that day. The judge also warned Golino that he would be held in contempt of court if he were involved in any further misconduct. Outside the courthouse, Golino told reporters that the prosecution feared him since he'd become an expert on the case and was sure that Grant was innocent.[10]

The following day, Dr. Carll Ladd, a lead criminalist in our DNA unit of the state police forensic sciences laboratory, testified on the DNA analysis from the bloodstains found at the crime scene. The odds, Ladd said, were 300 million to 1 that the blood samples were not those from Edward Grant. Dr. Ladd went on to testify that the state placed a 300-million-to-1 ceiling on its conservative calculation of the numbers, not wanting to prejudice a defendant with higher figures. Brian S. Carlow, an assistant defense counsel, challenged Dr. Ladd on the reliability of the DNA analysis, because of the age of those blood samples. Dr. Ladd was able to rely on many years of experience examining bloodstains. He concluded that the genetic profile of one individual could not mutate into the profile of another, no matter how old the bloodstain DNA evidence. The next day, world-renowned Yale University geneticist Professor Kenneth K. Kidd placed these DNA-matching figures at a much higher level. When asked by prosecutor James Clark for "the real number," Dr. Kidd set the odds at between 4.2 trillion and 6.1 trillion to 1, depending on the population database utilized. "I do not think it [the state's DNA ceiling number] correctly conveys how rare this profile is," Dr. Kidd said. The 4.2 to 6.1 trillion numbers would effectively cover the DNA of each and every human being who has ever lived on earth. The state's DNA ceiling figure, 300 million, would, of course, cover everyone living in the United States.[11] In reality, whether one in 300 million or one in 4.2 trillion, both calculations express the unique nature of the DNA in question. DNA results had a considerable impact on the court and the jurors in the outcome of the case.

I was called to testify on the morning of Thursday, May 9. Tom O'Neil, my coauthor, was in court that morning and noticed how the twelve jurors swung their focus toward me, as though they were students in a lecture hall. Even the defendant, Edward Grant, seemed to relax and to respond to my introduction. However, as Jim Clark began to question me on my reconstruction of the events on July 16, 1973, the defendant's expression seemed to harden considerably. The model of the Temple Street Garage sat a few feet directly in front of the jury box. I used the model to explain that our 1988 reconstruction of the events was based on a very careful review of police investigative records and the original crime scene photographs taken in 1973 on the day of the murder.

During my testimony, I described how the killer had chased Penney Serra, who was running barefoot through several levels of the garage. She ran into a dead-end at the base of the tenth-level stairwell and was stabbed in the heart there, only able to crawl to the third step where Penney fell and then crumpled into a fetal position at the base of the stairs, where she died.[12] Jim Clark, the prosecutor, at this juncture, exhibited a photo of Penney Serra's body lying in a fetal position at the base of the stairwell. I then explained to the jury the definition of a primary versus a secondary crime scene—that location where the murder actually occurred—and concluded that the garage fit that definition. I then explained how I thought the bloody latent fingerprints got onto the tissue box that was found on the floor behind the driver's seat of the Serra car. After running back to the lower level, the murderer got into the victim's car. He wanted to stanch the bleeding from a wound on his left hand, so he reached behind him as he started to drive the car through the garage. The tissue box must have been lying face down, so the murderer had to reach around the car's bucket seat to flip the box over in order to extract tissues to stop the bleeding. In this dynamic flipping motion, the assailant had left behind three bloody finger marks, due to direct contact, none of which yielded any readable ridges for fingerprint comparison. But in gripping the upright portion of the tissue box, the killer left the one clear fingerprint, his left thumbprint. Subsequent to this, the assailant also transferred some blood from his wound on top of this print. I added that was the most likely course of events, though, "I'm not saying that's the definite way, but the physical evidence indicates this was consistent with what happened."[13]

In his cross-examination, Tom Ullmann challenged the storage conditions of the white handkerchief found on the seventh level. Biological samples taken from it yielded the prosecution's DNA evidence, linking the blood to Grant. I explained how the blood-storage practices during the early days in the state police laboratory provided room temperatures that had adequately preserved the blood. Ullmann also asked how I could not provide a detailed positive link to the bloodied men's handkerchief found on the seventh level, about ten feet from the spot where Penney Serra's bloodied car keys were discovered, to the Serra car left on the eighth level, particularly since investigators never provided good photos of the blood trail. I affirmed that the investigators had not turned over a map of the garage or adequate photos of the blood trail. I said that I had to work with what I had been provided, telling the court that "I'm a pretty good cook, but if you don't give me rice or chicken or vegetables, I cannot make a meal." The defense counsel also stated that in my original 1988 reconstruction of the crime, I'd determined that there was "no direct linkage" between the handkerchief and the car. I replied that I'd modified my opinion when I had discovered that all of the blood DNA samples, from the car, from the blood trail, and from the handkerchief, had tested for type O. Later in the proceedings, James Clark would establish that, after rudimentary testing, a blood drop from the killer's trail matched Edward Grant's DNA profile. The twenty-nine years it took to bring this case to trial did produce one serious defect in the prosecution's case: somewhere along the line the bloodied white key ring and the keys to the Serra car found on the seventh level had been lost.

To back up its blood and DNA evidence, the prosecution next reached out to Dr. Edward Blake, a California geneticist in private practice who has provided valuable services for the Innocence Project—the New York–based organization that Barry Scheck, my colleague from the O. J. Simpson defense team, had played a key role in establishing. Blake, who worked full-time with Forensic Sciences Associates, has been instrumental in exonerating 108 falsely convicted defendants, using blood and forensic evidence. Dr. Blake testified the day after I had, and he placed the blood evidence from the garage at a "one in a trillion" chance that it was not Edward Grant's. In his cross-examination, assistant defense counsel Brian S. Carlow elicited from Blake testimony that DNA analysis cannot establish how long a blood sample has been on a surface or how it got there. Carlow also tried to establish a distinction between his own and the state's standards for establishing a match by a sample with a defendant's blood. Blake's terminology was that Grant was "included" as a source, while the state's term was that the defendant "could not be excluded." Dr. Blake dismissed this as "semantics," adding the question, "If I walk out of this courtroom and describe the sky as blue and someone else describes it as light blue, does that change the color of the sky?"[14] Following Dr. Blake, Inspector James Rouella from the district attorney's office testified that Edward Grant, shortly after his arrest, made the point that the railroad serial killer in Texas was caught "from a single fingerprint, too." In contrast to this self-incriminating evidence, Edward Grant's being fingerprinted as a result of charges that he beat his ex-fiancée was not allowed into evidence, since he was never convicted of those charges.[15]

Judge Blue had originally estimated that this trial would take somewhere between four and six weeks, and, as the prosecution moved on, it began to appear as though the case would go to the jury closer to the minimum. The following week, James Clark called Edward Grant's sister, Helene Thompson,* to the stand, who identified a 1973 photograph as one of Grant. It showed him sitting on a tow truck, with his arm around a family pet. The words "Wrecker Picture" appeared on the memo line of the check used to pay for the picture, which had been written there by one of her parents, Thompson said. Her parents had added the large wrecker to their business in the early seventies and wanted each family member to be photographed with it since they were proud of this addition. The two teenaged eyewitnesses at the Temple Street Garage on the day of the murder had provided police artists with enough information later that day to complete two sketches of the suspect. Both of these, when displayed, looked remarkably like the image displayed on the court's big screen of twenty-nine-year-old Edward Grant sitting on his family's new wrecker. Caesar Giori, a maintenance director at the Temple Street Garage, came to the stand and testified that he was just out of the hospital on the day of the murder and wasn't at work that day. This was significant since earlier statements made by garage employees on the day of the murder held that Giori had ordered a bloody palm print wiped off of a parking authority Jeep parked on the garage's tenth level.[16]

The prosecution finished presenting its witnesses the next day. Just as a good athlete wants to go to his greatest strength at a critical moment in a match, James Clark called Christopher Grice, a state expert on latent fingerprints, to testify on the latent print found on the tissue box. Comparing this critical piece of evidence with the fingerprint card rolled at the Waterbury police headquarters in 1994 by Edward Grant, Grice said that the tissue box print "came from the same person who left his left thumbprint on the ink card." Grice had been my student in the forensic science program at the University of New Haven in 1979. Upon his graduation, Grice joined the New Haven Police Department and was assigned to the ID unit in 1983, when he first examined the left thumbprint left on the tissue box. He had memorized its characteristics, its unique right angles and curves, and pointed out on the court's big screen the twelve ridge characteristics where the print matched the ink print taken from Edward Grant. This matching of ridge characteristics meant that the two prints matched "to the exclusion of all other people." This correlation was made in 1997. Under cross-examination by assistant public defender Beth Merkin, Grice said that there were other fingerprints in evidence that were examined and that were "not identifiable." In addition, he also pointed out that it was impossible to establish when, how, or why the left thumbprint matching Edward Grant's got on the tissue box. Beth Merkin argued that "as we sit here today, there are several prints that were lifted from the crime scene that we don't know whom they belong to." Grice agreed.

Following Grice's appearance, the prosecution and defense clashed over the expected appearance by a defense fingerprint expert. After Judge Blue had excused the jury, prosecutor Jim Clark argued that the defense was planning to introduce him to attempt to date the time that the blood droplet had spattered over the left thumbprint on the tissue box. Clark called this "junk science,"[17] adding that the defense knew that this determination could not scientifically be established. Chief defense counsel Tom Ullmann argued that the testimony would establish that the print was placed on the tissue box sometime before a blood drop spattered onto it. In my prior testimony, I had observed that the latent thumbprint was placed on the tissue box and that the blood smear could have been deposited on the box right after the print. The witness thus was not needed to testify, both sides would later concede.

During the midday of Thursday, May 16, Judge Blue led the jury, seven marshals, a court stenographer, and the prosecution and defense teams on a tour of the Temple Street Garage and the crime scenes. He did this, he said, for the jurors to get a better idea of what was being charged. Judge Blue displayed his sense of humor and his grasp of common sense by invoking the New York Yankee legend Yogi Berra, when he instructed the jurors how they should best take the tour: "You can observe a lot just by watching." The tour covered the two levels through which the prosecution charged that Edward Grant had chased his victim, finally stabbing her at the base of the tenth-level stairwell. They then passed through the six levels of the assailant's exit trail, including the spot on the eighth level where the suspect had erratically parked Penney Serra's Buick. They simultaneously listened to the appropriate portions of the prosecution's testimony. Orange cones marked critical spots throughout. The jurors were solemn and seemed to treat the base of the tenth-level stairwell where the victim's body was found as a shrine. Some became emotional and bit their lips. The jurors broke their tension and chuckled when the tour approached the spot where Bill Swanson had said he'd seen a man chasing Penney Serra, just after he'd gotten stoned with some friends on marijuana. Edward Grant's daughter accompanied the defendant on the tour.

Even though it was May, the weather this day was quite warm, though not as hot and muggy as on the date of the murder in 1973, partially due to a breeze that moved through the open-air garage. Several of the jurors asked Judge Blue to have someone stand at the spot where the investigators said the fatal chase began, but the judge declined, explaining that "there's no way of reproducing what was seen on July 16, 1973. It would be misleading rather than informative." *New Haven Register* reporter Christa Lee Rock later wrote that she had found the whole experience "eerie," like visiting the abandoned set of an old movie. She concluded her excellent article by noting that the tour finished right after 1:00 PM, just about the time the murder had occurred on that Friday, nearly thirty years earlier.[18] The prosecution did not call any witnesses to explain the motive behind the murder of Penney Serra.

The defense opened its case the first Monday afternoon following the tour. Bill Swanson's name had been on the defense's list of witnesses for that afternoon, but it was pulled, and he was never called. The defense's case was also marked by a second, far more significant, omission. Witnesses in Vermont affirmed the fact that Edward Grant had been there during the aftermath of floods that had been caused by heavy summer rains. However, further investigation by the prosecution indicated that the floods had occurred later in the summer, during the first part of August, and, thus, Grant's being there during that period was of no use to the defense as an alibi.[19] Still, Grant's defense team proved very energetic and resourceful as the trial moved into the following week. Tom Ullmann attacked the prosecution's inability to explain the unknown male DNA found in the crotch area of the victim's underpants and half-slip. Kathryn Colombo, a scientist with Orchid Cellmark of Maryland, testified that when she first examined the victim's underwear, she had found no evidence of sperm. However, after she had performed DNA tests, Colombo testified that she had been able to find Penney Serra's genetic markers mixed with traces of the Y chromosome DNA. Colombo said this finding could mean that the sperm was once on the garment, but had broken down, leaving only the trace Y chromosomal DNA she'd discovered. Colombo then added that this breakdown could have been caused by "environmental variables. DNA samples are best preserved in a cool, dry environment."[20]

Colombo's testimony directly followed that of William Paetzold, a former employee of the Connecticut Forensic Sciences Laboratory who later became a defense lawyer. Paetzold testified that the physical evidence from the Penney Serra case was stored for years at the lab's "transformer room," a space that was very hot. So much so, he said, that during the winter employees working outside often went into that room to warm themselves. Under cross-examination, the prosecution established that Paetzold had no experience with nor knowledge of DNA evidence. James Clark also established that, in 1973, detectives often did preliminary examinations of the presence of dried semen stains by merely running their fingers across a garment, feeling for a crusty substance. In his questioning, defense lawyer Brian Carlow countered that the prosecution could not explain how the Y chromosomal DNA had gotten onto these garments, thus leaving a gaping hole in their account of what had happened. Dr. Kimberlyn Nelson, a DNA expert from Mitotyping Technologies of Pennsylvania, then testified that she had conducted mitochondrial DNA tests on three nasal hairs found in the handkerchief, but her results were "inconclusive." Dr. Nelson explained that six key factors had to be examined. Edward Grant matched these specimens in five points. If the defendant did not match four or fewer points, then Dr. Nelson could have excluded him as a source, and if he had matched at all six points, the expert could have included Grant as a possible source for the hairs.[21]

As the trial of Edward Grant moved into its third full week, the defense called Edward Grant's first wife, Andrea Young,* to the stand. The couple had divorced in 1979. This witness established the fact that Grant always went to work wearing dark blue pants and a work shirt, not in the green pants and polo shirt that witnesses at the Temple Street parking garage said Penney Serra's assailant was wearing. Young also contradicted the testimony of Grant's sister, Helene Thompson, who, as a prosecution witness, had told the court that her brother always carried a white handkerchief with him. Young added that she would have noted white handkerchiefs while she'd washed her ex-husband's clothing, but never remembered seeing any there.[22]

The defense rested its case on the following day. During final arguments, James Clark laid out the prosecution's blood and fingerprint evidence in a step-by-step fashion. On the subject of motive, Clark said that Grant might have been attempting to steal the Serras' car and had killed his victim when she resisted. The defense team would later object to Clark's speculating on motive during the closing argument. In his own closing argument, defense counsel Thomas Ullmann urged the jurors to consider the physical condition of the blood evidence and how its deterioration over the years had compromised its validity as evidence. He also questioned whether the white handkerchief could have, instead, been part of a shirt. Ullmann also listed the trail of suspects police had investigated and had finally discarded over the course of twenty-nine years. Attorney Ullmann concluded his side's closing argument by asking that the jurors "return Eddy Grant to his family, where he belongs."[23]

Judge Blue, in his final charge to the jury, declared that the six men and six women had better get some rest in the following two days, "because you'll be working hard on Wednesday," when their deliberations would begin. He called the crime "one of the most mysterious murder cases in New Haven's history." Both sides had agreed to have Judge Blue instruct the jury that their verdict could be for a lesser offense, a conviction for manslaughter, if they felt that the defendant had not meant to kill Penney Serra but only to inflict "serious physical injury." This was very relevant since the penalty for murder was twenty-five to sixty years, and for manslaughter, it was ten to twenty-five years. This was an especially critical distinction, since no evidence on motive was ever introduced into evidence at this trial. In his ninety-minute summation, James Clark quoted testimony from Rosemary Serra on her sister's character: "Penney would have been tenacious."

The prosecution and defense teams had argued their cases very forcefully. Ever the diplomat, Judge Blue called both sides' closing arguments "magnificent." After hearing his instructions, the twelve jurors filed out of the courtroom just after 3:30 PM, Wednesday, May 22, to begin their deliberations.[24] By Friday there were indications that the jury was having trouble. During a mid-afternoon break, several jurors were observed splitting off from the others, and earlier in the day shouting was heard from inside their deliberation room. During the day, jurors reheard two pieces of police testimony. The first pertained to how the witness Bill Swanson had made eye contact with the early prime suspect Philip DeLieto and how it tainted Swanson's then identifying him as the assailant, out of eight individuals in the lineup. The second testimony was about the two dental invoices for Martin Cooratal found in the Serra car. At the close of business on that Friday, Judge Blue excused the tired-looking jurors for the long Memorial Day weekend, reminding them to avoid any and all news accounts on the case and to refrain from discussing the case with anyone.[25]

When the jury renewed its deliberations the following Tuesday, May 28, some courthouse veterans wondered out loud about how many more days would be needed for those twelve individuals to reach a unanimous decision. Perhaps the deliberations were leading to a jury deadlock, which could mean a mistrial. In midafternoon, however, all of this speculation abruptly ended when word spread through the New Haven courthouse's sixth floor that the jury had reached its verdict and would shortly be announcing its decision, ending the twenty days of trial. When the proceedings were reopened, Judge Jon Blue cautioned those in the room against emotional outbursts at the end of what he called "this long, drawn-out, high-stakes trial." Most in attendance seemed to be there for the Serra family. Finally, the foreman of the jury was called upon to read the verdict, and this verdict was "guilty" to the charge of murder in the first degree. When the guilty verdict was announced, the room seemed to breathe a collective sigh of relief. Edward Grant seemed to stagger when he heard of his conviction, and defense counsel Brian Carlow felt compelled to put his arms around his client to hold him up. Grant's wife, Linda, openly wept. Rosemary Serra, with tears flowing down her cheeks, reached across the barrier separating spectators from the trial's participants and exchanged a hug with the lead prosecutor, James Clark. Judge Blue ordered Grant held without bail, pending sentencing, which was initially set for August 16.[26]

Reflecting the courtroom's reaction to the verdict, the entire New Haven area seemed to be relieved. The next day's *New Haven Register* carried a single word in bold face at the top of page one, guilty. The photo below showed a jubilant Rosemary Serra walking down the courthouse steps, arm in arm with Jim Clark. The state's three major network television channels each led their evening news program with the verdict and a wrap-up of the trial. Thomas Ullmann immediately announced that the defense would be appealing the decision on several grounds, one of which was the prosecutor's speculation in his closing argument about the murder happening when Edward Grant tried to steal the Serra family Buick. Another reason for an appeal would be to challenge Judge Blue's not instructing the jury to take note of the prosecution's losing some of the evidence. Jurors interviewed said that their decision hinged directly on the DNA and fingerprint evidence. One juror said it was "the evidence—all of it. We did what we had to do. We had nowhere else we could go." Ironically, Jack DeLieto, Philip DeLieto's older brother, told a reporter that the decision came down on his late father's birthday. Until his death, Mr. DeLieto had yearned to see the case solved and his son finally exonerated in the eyes of so many in the area who still suspected Philip.[27]

Rosemary Serra also spoke that afternoon about her own late father. John Serra's advertisements in the papers had at first embarrassed and bothered her, she said. Only after Mr. Serra had died in late 1998, had Rosemary realized that she felt the responsibility to pick up her father's banner and to press on for justice for her beloved older sister. After the trial, Rosemary said, "I think she [Penney] is at peace, as well as my father. Because they know that I'm OK and that I've made it through. This part of my life is over. . . . After this many years, my family can finally rest in peace. My father had faith in the system and I can, too." Rosemary Serra then left the courthouse steps and went to her sister's grave in St. Lawrence Cemetery in West Haven, to give thanks for the trial's outcome. Gary Nicholson, an assistant prosecutor who worked closely with James Clark, summed things up when he said, "Everybody worked hard, the jury did as well, and they came up with the right decision."[28]

Like many other aspects of this case, the twenty-nine-year delay in its being brought to justice complicated the judge's sentencing decision. Under the original statutes, murder called for a sentence of twenty-five years to life, but the judge had the latitude of sentencing the convicted man to less. Under the current laws, Judge Blue would have to sentence Edward Grant to at least twenty-five years in prison, a sentence that had to be fully served. After a review, Judge Blue ultimately would be allowed the wider scope in sentencing under the 1973 statutes, with a minimum sentence of ten years to twenty-five years available to him. Because both sides had heavy workloads, the judge then granted delays in the case's sentencing, finally settling on Friday, September 27, 2002. That early-autumn day dawned bright and sunny. Judge Blue listened as character witnesses testified on behalf of Edward Grant, whereas Rosemary Serra talked about what her sister's murder had meant to her father and herself: "No prison sentence can quantify the living nightmare I have lived. How could someone leave my sister alone to die?" Grant took the stand in his own behalf and denied that he had murdered Penney Serra. That being said, he expressed his remorse for all of the pain and suffering the Serra family had been through. He then said, "However, the jury has convicted me and I ask for leniency. I lived my entire life trying to make life better for my family."

With the preliminary statements on the record, Judge Blue then announced his decision. His voice went up an octave, and his body seemed to thrust forward: "No one can deny that someone killed Penney Serra and thrust a knife in her heart. Someone left that beautiful young woman dead or dying in a dirty stairwell in a parking garage. No one can deny what the evidence shows beyond any doubt—that someone was you." Raising his voice still further, the judge called out a line from Shakespeare's tragedy Macbeth: "All of the perfumes of Arabia will not sweeten your bloodstained hands." Then Judge Blue sentenced Grant to a twenty-years-to-life term in prison for his crime of murder. After the sentencing, Thomas Ullmann again expressed the defense's disappointment at the trial's outcome and called the day's testimony "a charade," since, he said, Judge Blue had already made up his mind. Grant was led away by marshals. Rosemary Serra's image again graced page one of the New Haven Register, as she exchanged a hug with a female friend. Prosecutor James Clark, who had repeatedly referred to the murder as "a stranger crime" (meaning a crime against a stranger), boiled matters down after the sentencing when he said, "This case has to do with the Serra family, the detectives who did such a great job that day [July 16, 1973], and the technology."[29]

THE SUMMARY

Penney Serra's younger sister, Rosemary, summed up my feelings very eloquently after Grant's sentencing. "If you [Edward Grant] had come forward twenty-nine years ago, maybe I would not have had to look into my father's haunted eyes. You turned time into our enemy. I've spent 70 percent of my life looking over my shoulder, wondering if some acquaintance could have been the murderer."[30]

As the adage states, "Justice delayed is justice denied." It is unspeakably sad that John Serra did not live to hear Judge Blue call out his sentence, effectively sending Edward Grant to prison for the rest of his life. Perhaps, in some small way, Mr. Serra could have found inner peace. Perhaps he would have been able to lose what his daughter called a haunted look in his eyes. Yet local and state police investigators and the forensic team in our state laboratory never lost hope that the killer would be brought to justice. Along with John Serra, our team never gave up. That is the absolute key to solving cold cases. The desire to stay the course, along with the ability to keep looking at the evidence with a fresh perspective. Never give up. And, with the forensic technological breakthroughs that are exploding all around us, be ready when the final piece of evidence is found that becomes the key to the puzzle.

CHAPTER TWO

THE SKAKEL-MOXLEY CASE

A MURDER ON MISCHIEF NIGHT

Some people simply cannot keep a secret. As it turns out, he's [Michael Skakel's] been talking about his night of mischief since at least the spring of 1978.
—Jonathan Benedict, Assistant State's Attorney, in trial's opening statement, May 7, 2002

Death is the natural culmination of life. We all know that the finality of death is inescapable. However, when the death is of a fifteen-year-old, innocent girl, a highly intelligent and beautiful young lady just moving into the full bloom of her young womanhood, then the death seems much more tragic. When this death is the result of murder, it is moreover a shock to the community. Martha Moxley of Greenwich, Connecticut, was just such a vital and promising teenaged girl when the breath of life was savagely beaten from her on the cold night of October 30, 1975, on the broad expanse of her family's suburban hillside yard.

Earlier on that dark and moonless evening, Martha's mother, Dorthy Moxley, had been busying herself painting window frames in her master bedroom. Her husband, David, the managing partner in the Manhattan offices of Touche, Ross, a Big Eight accounting firm, was away on business and would not be returning home until the next evening to celebrate his forty-fourth birthday with his family. As the evening progressed, Mrs. Moxley descended to the living room of her large Tudor-style home, where she dozed off, awaiting the early return of her daughter and that of her older child, John, seventeen. This was Mischief Night, so-called since it is the night before Halloween, when America's suburban children, on a rare school night out, often play pranks on neighbors, moving about in small packs, stringing toilet paper on trees and bushes. Before midnight, Dorthy Moxley was startled awake by the sound of someone entering her home. It was John, which surprised her, since he was home before his younger sister. Even before this moment, Mrs. Moxley had felt a vague sense of dread about her daughter's whereabouts. Now, fully awakened, she started to make calls to her neighbors and Martha's teenaged friends, waking them up in an effort to find her daughter. Indeed, just the previous weekend, Dorthy Moxley had severely reprimanded Martha for coming home after one in the morning, an unusual misdeed by the well-behaved teenager. Martha had then tried to laugh off her behavior, giving her mother a flimsy excuse on where and with whom she had been until that late hour. As Mischief Night moved several hours into the next day, Mrs. Moxley anxiously phoned more family friends and neighbors.

One of the very first calls Mrs. Moxley initially made was to the home of Rushton Skakel Sr., her next-door neighbor. Mr. Skakel, a widower for the past two years, was away in upper New England on a hunting trip. The two families lived two hundred yards apart on adjoining roads in the Belle Haven section of Greenwich—a gated, guarded, and exclusive part of the town, considered to be one of the most affluent in America. In her call to the Skakel home, Mrs. Moxley talked to Julie, eighteen, Mr. Skakel's only daughter and second oldest of seven children. Two of Julie's younger brothers,

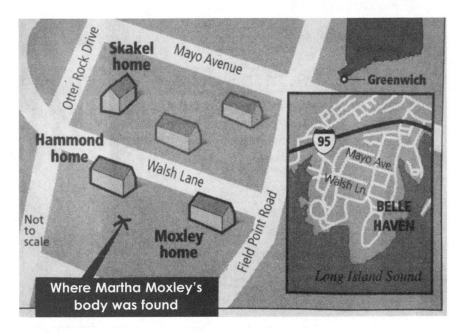

Maps and diagram of the crime scene.

Tom, seventeen, and Michael, fifteen, were friendly with Martha. Julie told Mrs. Moxley that she'd last seen Martha with her brother, Tom.[1]

Even in the privileged and exclusive world of Belle Haven, the Skakel family stood out as particularly wealthy. Rushton Skakel's younger sister, Ethel, was the widow of Sen. Robert F. Kennedy, the former attorney general of the United States and member of the United States Senate, and the younger brother of the late president John F. Kennedy. Both of the Kennedys had been assassinated while in office, and both were prominent members of one of the wealthiest and most politically powerful families in American history. Indeed, the Kennedy family, with its wealth and power, stood out then, as it does today, as a clan famous for its long line of personal tragedies, extending as far back as World War II, when Joseph, the oldest boy, was killed in action. Later in the war, the British husband of the eldest daughter, Kathleen, was killed in action when his RAF plane was shot down. Kathleen herself then died in a plane crash in

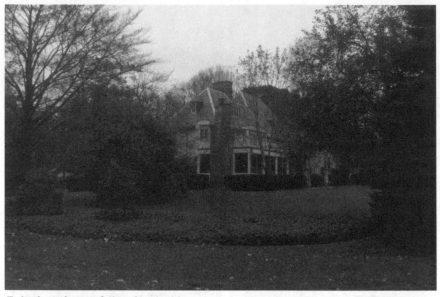

Exterior view of the Skakel house.

1948. Since Robert F. Kennedy's 1968 death, two of his sons have died; in addition, Jacqueline Kennedy Onassis died of cancer in 1994 at age sixty-five, and in the summer of 1996, John F. Kennedy Jr., his wife, and his sister-in-law all died in a plane crash off Martha's Vineyard.

Rushton Skakel himself was the scion of a family fortune at least as huge as that of the Kennedys. He headed Great Lakes Carbon, the privately owned mineral conglomerate that had pioneered the production of aluminum from coal and coke residue during the aircraft building boom of the thirties. And, like the enormously wealthy Kennedy clan, the Skakel family had already experienced a great deal of personal tragedy. Rushton's parents and his older brother, George Jr., had all died in plane crashes, leaving him in charge of Great Lakes Carbon and the Skakel family fortune.[2]

On that Mischief Night in 1975, Dorthy Moxley kept up her frantic phone calls for several more hours, and, finally, at 3:48 AM, she phoned the Greenwich Police Department. A patrolman was dispatched to talk with her and to look around the Belle Haven streets for Martha. By dawn, Martha Moxley was still not found. Dorthy Moxley, now fully alarmed, had concerned neighbors and friends over to her home. Some sat with her in her living room, and some moved about the Belle Haven grounds, looking for any trace of the missing teenager. Finally, in the early afternoon, Martha's partially clad corpse was discovered by one of her close friends, Colleen O'Dwyer,* on the Moxley property, lying face down under a large pine tree. Colleen, like several other teenagers, had joined police, firemen, and volunteers to search for Martha Moxley.

This horrible discovery set off shock waves that were immediate and far-reaching. The thirty or so members of the Greenwich Police Department had not investigated a complex homicide in many years, and now that suddenly changed. The national news media soon were drawn into this case, due in large part to the Skakel family's relationship to the Kennedy family. The crime also took on added significance since it took place in wealthy Greenwich, Connecticut, an exclusive and protected community that, unlike most of the rest of America, was supposedly free of horrific crimes like this one.[3]

From the outset of the investigation, several critical errors were made. Foremost was the failure to protect and preserve the crime scenes. Many unauthorized and nonessential individuals were allowed to move about the hillside on which Martha's body had been found and along the ground where her slayer had dragged her body. This all occurred before the police investigators could secure the crime scenes, greatly contaminating these critical venues. In subsequent months, the Greenwich police, despite assistance from the Connecticut State Police and the FBI, were not able to make an arrest or achieve any solution for this case. Over the years, of course, there was the growing suspicion that Martha Moxley's murderer was not found due to the Skakel family's enormous wealth and to political pressure applied by their powerful in-laws, the Kennedy family.

All of these factors led to the Moxley murder becoming an old and cold case, albeit one that periodically attracted intense national media attention. As the years became decades since the night of October 30, 1975, the Moxley family was left to mourn Martha's death without any sense of closure, let alone the satisfaction of seeing justice done. In the later seventies, the behaviors of several suspects in this case became important. The teenaged Michael Skakel's troubled life led his family to enroll him in an expensive school in Maine that specialized in dealing with individuals who had problems. Going back to the afternoon of the murder, a live-in tutor recently hired by Rushton Skakel reported to the Skakel residence to work with Tom and Michael. Bruce Atwell* moved into the family home, and he would soon fall under suspicion. In subsequent years, the police interest in Atwell skyrocketed because of his increasingly bizarre behaviors and his minor brushes with the law. Police suspicion of Atwell was compounded by his failing two polygraph tests that asked whether he killed Martha Moxley. Tom Skakel also took a polygraph test, which he failed to pass, though he did better in a second test given to him.[4]

In 1991 a special task force made up of members of the Bridgeport State's Attorney's office, the Greenwich Police Department, and the State Police Forensic Sciences Laboratory was formed to conduct a new review of the Moxley case, and I became a member of this ad hoc team. In 1999 the work of the task force led to the case being assigned to a one-man grand jury. Martha Moxley's murder would eventually become the case in which the legal community would learn to deal with the concept of "indirect forensic evidence," a term I used in the spring of 2001, when I testified at the case's murder trial. (Later on in this chapter, I will detail what is meant by this concept.)

Central to this case was Michael Skakel's telling fellow students and staff at Maine's Elan School that he had murdered Martha Moxley. I will delve into the subject of confessions, once considered the "silver bullet" of a prosecution's case. I will also explore the use of lie detector tests and why they are considered inadmissible in courts of law. The Moxley murder ultimately sheds light on the solution of cold cases through teamwork, as well as the absolutely essential need for investigators to present the whole truth and nothing but the truth, as they are best able to do, no matter the consequences, no matter who is ultimately involved, and no matter what jurisdictional boundaries have to be crossed.

THE FACTS OF THE CASE

To gain a fuller perspective on this case, it helps to know the history regarding the two families: the Skakels and the Moxleys. Dorthy Moxley and her husband, David, were both products of the Midwest. Dorthy Jolgren was born in 1932 in Iron River, Michigan, up north near the Wisconsin border, the only daughter of a Finnish father and a Swedish mother. When she was four, her parents moved her and an older brother to Rochester, Michigan, so that Mr. Jolgren, a tool and die maker, could work in the auto industry's thriving plants, primarily for Dodge and also for naval ordnance during World War II. Dorthy's family settled into an older wooden home, one that initially had no indoor plumbing. Dorthy's father, John Jolgren, an indefatigable worker, was able to remedy this problem and continued to add on to his home, as well as to surround the family with all manner of fruit trees. Dorthy's mother, Emma Lundvald Jolgren, matched her husband's industrious nature by keeping their home spotless. As was the custom in those Depression years, Dorthy would walk a mile along a gravel road to school. When she was in the second grade, Dorthy's best friend was run over and killed by one of the huge gravel trucks that rumbled up and down the narrow road. This would be her first encounter with violent death. Much of the information on the Moxley and Skakel family backgrounds, as well as many of the case's early details, are spelled out in the excellent book *Greentown: Murder and Mystery in Greenwich, America's Wealthiest Community*, written by Timothy Dumas.[5]

Aside from this childhood tragedy, Dorthy's growth into young womanhood was a classic example of American families coping with and finding happiness during the Great Depression and the harrowing years of World War II. Dorthy was a good student and later became a cheerleader at Rochester High School. She was voted the most popular girl in her class. After graduation, Dorthy gained admission to Michigan State University in East Lansing, just as that huge school was climbing out from under the shadow of the state's first university at Ann Arbor. With Michigan State's admission to the prestigious Big Ten athletic conference, the school's football team won the conference championship and the right to play in the annual Rose Bowl game in 1955, a trip Dorthy didn't make. This was an event, nonetheless, that would change her life forever. Dorthy was enchanted by the tales of California sunshine and palm trees, stories told by a sorority sister who had made the Rose Bowl trip, so that's where she and three other girlfriends headed after graduation the following spring.

Dorthy had majored in education, and she was able to land a job teaching the fifth grade at a public school in Long Beach. At that time, many recent college grads went into the military service as officers, products of the Reserve Officer Training programs that dotted the American collegiate landscape. On one evening, Dorthy and her friends met a junior naval officer from a nearby shore station, David Moxley, who hailed from Atchison, Kansas, where his father was an assistant postmaster. As often happens when groups of people meet, one of Dorthy's girlfriends developed a quick crush on David, whom Dorthy found nice but not particularly attractive. At her friend's urging, Dorthy had long talks with David to get all of the facts on him. After a while, though, the couple found they were falling in love and announced their engagement the following New Year's Eve. They were married in a military wedding the following March and moved back to Lawrence, Kansas, when David's two-year service requirement ended. There Dorthy found a job teaching school, supporting her husband while he got his MBA at the University of Kansas, financing his studies under the GI Bill. David was an excellent student. He graduated in 1958 with honors and later passed his first CPA test. Touche, Ross & Company, the prestigious accounting firm, then offered David a job in San Francisco. Dorthy, five months pregnant, and her husband found themselves back in California. Their first child, John, was born the following October, and Martha rounded out the family in 1960. In 1962 they bought a modest house north of Oakland in the Bay area. In the next twelve years, David Moxley worked very hard, spending many long evening hours at the offices of Kaiser, a key corporate client. This meant, just as with his studies back at Lawrence, Kansas, that David was out of the home for long periods of time. This also resulted in his gaining national notice at Touche, Ross, which eventually, in 1974, offered David the managing partner's job at the firm's flagship office in New York City, an offer he proudly accepted.[6]

Coming east in 1974, the Moxley family's decision to purchase a home in Greenwich's exclusive Belle Haven section was both affordable and pragmatic, given David's new position. As the top administrator for Touche, Ross's headquarters in Manhattan, David Moxley would be commanding a base salary well into six figures, plus his bonuses and the other add-ons that go with such a prestigious job. The daily trips to the city, whether by a commuter train, which made runs around the clock, or by car, would normally take less than an hour. Their new state did not have its own income tax, as did neighboring New York and New Jersey, and that would save a considerable amount of money. The Greenwich public school system was considered among the very best in the country. This would also save the Moxley family the cost of private schooling. Thus, the entire family moved into picturesque Greenwich and its privileged life with great enthusiasm and with the prospects for many happy and fulfilling years ahead of them.

Like the Moxleys, the Skakel family came to Greenwich from its roots in America's heartland. George Skakel Sr. had founded Great Lakes Coal & Coke Company with two partners in 1919. A natural-born entrepreneur, the elder Skakel had bought out his two associates and soon found himself in sole control of a gold mine. The dusty tons of coke that George's company had been buying cheaply and removing from the properties of the country's big petroleum refineries was a natural, if unwanted, residue of the process of creating gasoline. Skakel, with the help of a hefty bank loan, was able to all but corner the market on this coke, which he then distilled into carbon, a substance essential to the production of aluminum. All this was happening at the same time that the American aircraft industry, spurred on by Charles Lindbergh, was swinging into the mass production of aircraft made of aluminum.

In 1934 George and Ann Skakel purchased a mansion in what the people of Greenwich like to call its "back country," located north of the Post Road, the Merritt Parkway, and the route that would later become the Connecticut Turnpike. The couple purchased this home surrounded by an estate full of woods and grounds with winding gravel pathways and fountains from the Simmons family, originators of the still-successful mattress company, for $100,000, an enormous price for that time. Ann Skakel was a devout Roman Catholic and as the mother insisted that her seven children be baptized and raised in her faith, as was the custom for "mixed marriages" of that day. The Skakel children all attended private schools, and the four girls all were sent to exclusive Catholic colleges, such as Manhattanville College, just across the New York border in Purchase. Two of the three Skakel boys quickly gained a local reputation as hell-raisers, though Rushton, the youngest, did not. In 1945, her first year at Manhattanville, Ethel Skakel met Jean Kennedy, the daughter of Joseph Kennedy, the former United States ambassador to Great Britain and a megamillionaire in his own right. Thus, the two large Catholic families began to socialize, and Ethel eventually married Robert F. Kennedy at St. Mary Church in Greenwich on June 17, 1950.

In the next two decades, tragedy struck the Skakel family. Ann and George Skakel were killed in a plane crash in Oklahoma in 1955. Then, in 1966, their son George Jr. was killed in the crash of a small plane while on an elk-hunting trip in Idaho. On a balmy Thanksgiving afternoon later that year, George's oldest daughter, Kick, a teenager, took neighborhood children on a ride in a new family car, and a six-year-old girl was accidentally thrown from her perch on top of the convertible's backseat and subsequently died of her injuries. Later on, George's widow, Pat, choked to death on a piece of meat at a family dinner party. George's death in the midsixties had led to his brother Rushton Skakel becoming the chief executive officer of Great Lakes Carbon, as the gigantic corporation had become known. Unlike his deceased older brother, Rushton Skakel was not an overly assertive individual. Quiet, pleasant, and unassuming by nature, he did not seem to relish this new and heavy responsibility. Rushton also had problems with drinking, problems so severe that, by today's standards, he would have to be categorized as an alcoholic. This all meant that the Skakel family fortune would diminish, though its size would still be measured by many millions of dollars.[7]

In the later sixties, Rushton's wife, Ann Reynolds Skakel, was diagnosed with cancer. The mother of the seven Skakel children fought a brave battle with this disease. For years Ann Skakel seemed to be surviving, but in 1972 her condition worsened, and she died in 1973. This left Rushton Sr. with six boys and one girl, aged from seven to seventeen years old. Even with a family fortune at his disposal, this tragic turn of events seemed, by all accounts, to be too much for Rushton Skakel to handle, and he increasingly relied on alcohol as his escape. Rushton also had his physical escapes and seemed to neighbors and friends to be away from home an inordinate amount of time, on hunting and other pleasure trips or on business trips. Household staff, such as a maid, teachers and officials at the private schools the children all attended, or the several priests who visited regularly were the only adults to provide any semblance of order and discipline for the Skakel children. On many evenings some or all of the siblings would walk a few hundred yards down to the Belle Haven Club on Long Island Sound, where they would be served dinner and, on many occasions, alcoholic beverages.

Belle Haven neighbors worried about the Skakel children. Since Ann Skakel's death, it seemed obvious to them that things were often out of hand in the family's huge house. Unsupervised parties and late-night gatherings of teenaged kids were the order of the day. Parents worried about how this all would impact their own children. Dorthy Moxley was apprehensive about her teenaged son and daughter being drawn into the bacchanals, particularly Martha, who had blossomed into a beautiful young lady. Yet Dorthy still felt sympathetic toward these children for having lost their mother and for the way things were drifting so badly out of hand. And Dorthy Moxley didn't have the whole picture. When he was just four, Tommy Skakel had suffered a traumatic brain injury that left him unconscious for many hours. This could possibly account for his later behavior, such as violent outbursts—horrible episodes that often led to severe physical punishment from his father or from some other adult. Michael, two years younger, seemed to emulate Tom, and the two had what can be called an intense love-hate relationship. Like other male siblings close in age and body size, Tom and Michael regularly fought each other.

*   *   *

For many families, a three-thousand-mile summer move out of northern California to aloof Greenwich would have proven a monumental challenge. But not to the Moxley family. Starting with Martha's first few days as an incoming freshman at Greenwich High School, she was immediately accepted. She had long, blond hair, which she parted directly in the middle, a fashion of the midseventies, and her new schoolmates quickly took to her, both the girls and the boys. At the end of her freshman year, Martha was even elected the most popular student in her class. Dorthy and David Moxley were quickly recognized as talented and pleasant people, good neighbors, not at all the stereotype of fast-lane California folk. John, Martha's older brother, also did not have any trouble making new friends in his junior class at the public high school. Closer to home, in Belle Haven, where they'd moved into a large and comfortable house, the Moxley children met and became acquainted with their neighbors, the Skakel children, who did not go to their high school, but to a private school, instead.[8]

But it was Martha, in particular, who thrived in her new East Coast environment. Her good looks only improved when the braces on her teeth were removed, enhancing her already lovely and wide smile. Michael Skakel, her neighbor from around the corner on Otter Rock Drive, was the first of the Skakel family's boys to get to know Martha. In late spring, his name appeared in an entry in the diary that Martha diligently added to every few days. Michael was also, according to observers, the better looking of the two rival Skakel brothers. During the course of the summer, however, Martha also became acquainted with Michael's older brother, Tommy, and wrote approvingly of him. In contrast, Michael, perhaps because of his reputation for bizarre behavior, such as his firing an air rifle at neighborhood pets, later got some bad ink in Martha's notes to herself. But Martha found a boyfriend away from her Belle Haven neighborhood, a nice-looking classmate from her high school who was proud that he had beaten out the sons of a powerful businessman for her affections. The summer of 1975 meant a return to peacetime for America, since the last military forces had been pulled out of Vietnam the previous spring. And in her fifteenth summer, Martha Moxley and her circle of girlfriends basked in the beauty of their storybook surroundings. A half-dozen or so of the girls enjoyed going "pool-hopping," suddenly showing up at someone's swimming pool, splashing around noisily, and finishing their impromptu and uninvited visit with loud cannonball dives. Martha remained light-hearted and happy with her new friends, surroundings, family, and life.

In the fall of the 1975 Rushton Skakel decided to hire Bruce Atwell, a broad-shouldered young man of twenty-three who had been recommended by the headmaster of a local private school where Bruce taught. This was due to the poor grades that his two middle sons, Tom and Michael, had been receiving. Rushton Skakel had hoped Atwell would be a good role model for his two sons, as well as their tutor. Atwell moved into the Skakel home in the middle of the afternoon of Thursday, October 30.

As the end of October approached, Dorthy Moxley had forgiven her daughter for her late and unexplained return home the previous weekend. Martha was thus given permission to host a party for her friends the following Friday night, Halloween. The family decorated their downstairs recreation room for the expected festivities. Martha had also arranged a date for her neighbor and close friend, Colleen O'Dwyer, for Thursday night. Colleen, who was as shy with boys as Martha was outgoing, had a secret crush on a particular boy for quite some time, and the two girls looked forward to sharing a full accounting of the date on the way to school the next morning. As she went about her evening, Colleen thought that Martha was planning to go out of Belle Haven and over to her boyfriend's house to help cook dinner.

That moonless Mischief Night of 1975 proved cold. It was cold enough for people to see their exhaled breath. This cold, of course, would not deter the area's youth in bringing mischief and not a little mayhem to the adult community. In Belle Haven, the grown-ups expected this and, through their association, had hired a special policeman to protect their property on Mischief Night. This was in addition to the twenty-four-hour-a-day guard at the entrance to their enclave on Long Island Sound. The special guard, Anthony Whelan,* was more than ready for his assignment; he was a veteran of two and a half years in Vietnam. Yet, when Whelan left the Belle Haven Club to go about his job, an inexplicable feeling of dread came over him. Whelan first spotted a speed fence that a car had knocked over. He got out of his car to put it back up. Around nine, he observed a larg- ish group of teenagers, a dozen or so, under some trees on the Moxley property. He approached the group, who noticed him, and, as kids will do, they all rapidly ran off. They ran in the direction of the Skakel house on Otter Rock Drive. A little later on, Whelan saw a large, bespectacled, and blond young man walking down Walsh Lane, and, since this individual looked out of place, he asked him what he was doing there. The man identified himself as a neighbor who was simply out for a walk. Later on, Whelan saw the same man at a distance, disappearing between two houses.[9]

The guard's evening had started with a visit to the Belle Haven Club where he was able to scrounge a hot cup of coffee from the kitchen help. Newly appointed tutor Bruce Atwell also showed up at the club, since all of the Skakel children, plus a cousin and a girl- friend of Julie Skakel's, had dinner there that night, with their new boarder as guest. Michael Skakel ordered and consumed more than one rum and coke, even though he was only fifteen. Atwell didn't stop him. Besides getting a buzz on, Michael was already at work testing his boundaries with his new disciplinarian. Michael's cousin Jimmy Terrien, whose mother, Georgeann, was Rushton Skakel's sister, was also a Skakel family guest for dinner at the club that night.

After their dinner at the club, the Skakel party dispersed. Julie returned home to do some homework, watch television, and, in general, keep an eye on her younger brothers. This role of surrogate parent had fallen to her since her mother's death. Around 9:30 PM, the youngest child, Steven, age nine, was awakened by a loud argu- ment coming from his yard, with people screaming at one another. He went back to sleep. On this Mischief Night, one twelve-year-old boy in the neighborhood thought he heard heavy footsteps in the thick leaves that covered much of the ground. He ran back home. Another twelve-year-old boy was awakened by what sounded like people screaming. An adult neighbor, a man who would later rise in the ranks of New York City prosecutors, let his springer spaniel out to relieve itself before coming in for the night. Instead of coming back to the house, he saw the dog disappear from view. Worried, the man stood and called for the dog, to no avail. He went back in the house for a time and then returned to find his dog, looking chastened, returning to his house from the direction of the Moxley house. The man was convinced that the dog was upset and was trying to tell him something. A married couple heard what they thought was a dog growling. A twelve-year-old girl, who was in bed, heard her family's German shepherd barking excitedly around 10:00 PM. She went downstairs to the back door to see why her dog was so upset, only to be sent back upstairs by a maid.

At about the same time and from her vantage point in her bedroom upstairs, Dorthy Moxley heard what she would later call some kind of "commotion" going on below her window. There was the sound of two or three male voices in a loud argument. Dorthy debated going downstairs to turn on the outside lights, but decided against it since she worried that some mischief-maker might find Martha's new, ten-speed, bright yellow Schwinn bike and decide to take it. The sounds from outside subsided, and Dorthy returned to a chore, some painting. At the Skakel house, a maid had also heard some discord from outside, and she called up to Bruce Atwell, who was watching the movie *The French Connection* on the master bedroom's television. She asked him to come down and check on what was causing the disturbance. Atwell descended, opened the front door, looked around, and heard some rustling in the leaves. Seeing nothing, he returned upstairs to his movie. Around 11:00 PM, a twenty-three-year-old neighbor who lived across the street from the Skakel home and three lots away from the Moxley house thought he heard something coming from the Moxleys' end of Walsh Lane. He turned out the light and went to bed. The wind had picked up, making the chilly night even chillier.[10]

Colleen O'Dwyer returned home from her date shortly before midnight. Disappointed with how things went, she hoped that Martha would cheer her up in the morning. Colleen went up the driveway to the front door of her home, only to find it locked. Cold and with no key, she tried throwing stones at the upstairs windows to awaken someone to let her in. Nobody awakened, and Colleen then decided to go into the garage and get into the family car to warm herself. The cold air quickly penetrated her retreat. Colleen then heard what sounded like a door creak, perhaps from the potting shed behind the garage. She didn't want to find out what caused this sound, so she again threw stones at the upstairs windows. Soon her mother came down and let her cold daughter into the house. At the Moxley household, Dorthy had been waiting in vain for Martha's return home. She dozed off in the living room and was awakened around 11:20 PM by her older child, John, who had returned from a night out with two of his friends. John's arrival, far from reassuring Mrs. Moxley, unsettled the apprehensive parent further. John almost always came home after his kid sister. John agreed to look for Martha and drove about Belle Haven and Greenwich for a half hour without any luck.

Dorthy Moxley then became deeply concerned about her daughter's whereabouts. She started making calls to as many of Martha's friends as she could think of and to her neighbors. Colleen O'Dwyer was awakened by Mrs. Moxley at 2:00 AM. Colleen said that she'd thought that Martha had planned to go to her boyfriend's house earlier in the evening. Mrs. Moxley was perplexed that Martha had changed her plans. Nearly two hours later, Colleen was again awakened by another call from the now-frantic Dorthy Moxley. Colleen thought that Martha had probably gone to somebody's house and had decided to sleep over there. At three in the morning, Dorthy Moxley awakened her son, and this time John shared his mother's fears. He drove back out in the family car to look for his sister, finally returning empty-handed, three hours later, at just about dawn. Finally, at 3:48 AM, Dorthy Moxley called the Greenwich Police Department to report that her daughter had been missing since the previous evening. A car was dispatched to the Moxley residence, and word on the missing girl was spread to other patrol cars.

Between the calls to Colleen, Mrs. Moxley called the Terrien household, in the northern section of Greenwich. Georgeann Terrien, Rush Skakel's sister, didn't know anything about Martha's whereabouts and was upset by the 3:00 AM call. Before going back to bed, she looked in her son Jimmy's bedroom, only to find that he wasn't there. Georgann surmised that her son must have stayed over at his cousins', the Skakels', house in Belle Haven, so she went back to sleep.

As the sun rose over the waters at the western end of Long Island Sound on the morning of October 31, very few people were aware that a fifteen-year-old girl was missing. The Greenwich police made sweeps through Belle Haven looking for Martha. During their response to Mrs. Moxley's 3:48 AM call, the officers had noticed the Halloween party decorations in the family room. This made them wonder why a youngster would risk her parents' anger just before she was allowed to throw a party. But, still, they must have conjectured, teenaged kids sometimes do the oddest things. As the morning became bright, sunny, and clear, the private-school children got ready for a regular Friday at school, while the public-school kids relished the thought of going in for only a half day, since there would be teacher conferences in the afternoon. Almost everyone went about their business as usual.

Early that morning, Dorthy Moxley awakened in her downstairs library. She quickly moved outside her house into the chilly air to look for her missing daughter. Her quest took her to the Skakel residence, where Michael answered the door, looking pale, his long, stringy hair wet. Dorthy Moxley introduced herself to the tired-looking teenager, since they had never talked before. No, Michael replied, he did not know where Martha might be. Dorthy noticed a tan camper parked in the Skakel driveway on the side of the house. Maybe Martha had fallen asleep there, perhaps after one too many beers. Mrs. Moxley and Michael asked the Skakel's gardener, Dennis Murdock,* to check out the camper, which he did. No Martha. Dorthy returned home, feeling very alone. Since her husband, David, was in Atlanta on a business trip, she telephoned him to alert him to Martha's absence. John Moxley ate his breakfast, and, though exhausted and worried himself, he went off to school on schedule.

Several concerned neighbors walked about Walsh Lane and the surrounding streets looking for any sign of Martha. As the morning dragged on, Dorthy was joined by several women, mothers of Martha's closest friends, and several Belle Haven neighbors. Dorthy told them how unlikely it was for her daughter not to come home or at least call. David Moxley called from Atlanta to find his daughter was still missing. In desperation, Dorthy Moxley again called the Greenwich police, who had nothing to report.

During her morning at school, Colleen O'Dwyer began to feel fear tighten its grip on her. She loved her best friend, and she shuddered as word began to spread through the school that Martha had been missing since the night before. Finally, since school had an early dismissal that day, Colleen set out on a mission to find Martha. As soon as she stepped down off of her bus in Belle Haven, she began systematically covering the grounds near her own home and those lying behind an ornate and high brick wall, near the Moxley and Skakel houses. She called out Martha's name as she looked. Colleen met another teenaged Belle Haven girl who helped her search for a while but then left. The other child was afraid of what might be found, though she did not express this macabre thought to Colleen. Finally, after about a half hour of searching, Colleen was moving up the gentle hillside on the Moxley property, with the house to her right, toward a majestic pine. She thought she saw some pink and blue camping gear under the green boughs, which were undulating to the dull and chill wind. As Colleen advanced, she was shocked to find her dear friend's partially clad, murdered body, lying face down. Colleen became almost catatonic as the reality of what she had discovered began to set in.

Years later, author Tim Dumas interviewed Colleen, who was able to describe the wounds to Martha's body that she first observed that day: Martha's feet were pointed up the slope, and her head was tilted toward her own house. Martha was wearing blue jeans, pulled down, along with her underpants, to the middle of her thighs. On her upper body, she had on a light blue, L.L. Bean–style down jacket that had a quilted surface. There were scratches and deep gouges on her hips, extending down to her thighs. The blood from these wounds had collected pine needles and other debris. Blood was also visible in her blond hair. What was visible of Martha's face appeared scratched and scraped. As best as Colleen was able to remember, her friend's arms were stretched down the slope, around her head.[11]

Back in the cold sunlight of that early afternoon in 1975, Colleen was able to gather enough strength to go to the Moxley home and blurt out her discovery of Martha, though she was unable or unwilling to say that she thought that her dear friend was dead. The women in the living room were all horrified. Dorthy Moxley, she remembered, was somehow able to contain herself, and the others wisely suggested that Colleen take Betty McCormick,* a neighbor, to where she had found Martha. The distraught teenager had the wherewithal to approach the pine tree, but not enough to go through what she had before. Fifty or so feet up the hillside from the pine tree, Colleen crumpled to her knees, weeping into her hands, as Betty moved farther down the hillside and under the tree's outstretched branches to Martha's side. She reached down quickly and made her grim assessment. Colleen and Betty then returned to the Moxley home, and Dorthy, who was sitting, did not look up, but simply asked: "Is she dead?" Betty waited a half second before telling Dorthy the horrible truth.[12]

THE INVESTIGATION OF THE CASE

Before getting directly into the Moxley investigation, I feel it is important to stress again the fact that in 1975 the Greenwich Police Department did not have much experience in dealing with a homicide of this magnitude. The force primarily worked to assure a smooth traffic flow in its upscale downtown district and to protect the considerable wealth and property found in its homes and in the commercial stores in its central business district. The Greenwich Police Department was, put quite simply, overmatched by the complexity of this homicide investigation. Compounding this problem was a breakdown in support for the local police by the state's medical examiner's office, a development that would impede this investigation for many years. And, moreover, there was the suggestion that two of the most likely suspects were from the Skakel family, with all its wealth and political connections, factors that had to intimidate law enforcement from the very moment that Martha Moxley's body was discovered.

To underscore these points, consider the background of the first two officers who responded to the first report of Martha Moxley's body being found at 12:30 PM that Friday: they were both officers from the department's juvenile division. This meant that they were not homicide detectives, but youth officers whose specialty was dealing with teenage crime. Careful not to divulge the nature of the call, the dispatcher asked the two men to respond by telephone, since any radio transmissions would be bound to attract unwanted public and, inevitably, media attention. The two juvenile officers raced to Belle Haven and to the Moxleys' front door, where they found the home full of women in tears. Directed outside, they located Martha's body and confirmed the murder. Their immediate response was that some maniac had bludgeoned the teenager to death. The officers quickly called for assistance, and they were soon joined by a captain and two detectives. The captain tried unsuccessfully to find a pulse. They all noted that rigor mortis had already set in as well as the discoloration of the body caused by the blood's settling due to gravity, which is termed *lividity*, or *livor mortis*.

At this time, a parade of outsiders began to arrive at the crime scene. One of the first of these was someone whose presence was valuable. One of Dorthy Moxley's neighbors had called in the Moxley family physician, who was persuaded to leave a lecture he'd been attending in downtown Greenwich. The police provided him access to Martha's body, where he noted that the major wound to her head was so severe that it had penetrated her skull, and he could actually see the gray matter of her brain. This doctor then proceeded into the house, where he spoke gently to Dorthy Moxley, who had been sitting immobile on her living-room couch. Just then the phone rang, and another neighbor answered a call from David Moxley. At first, this lady could only urge Mr. Moxley to come home at once, until, under persistent and pointed questioning by David, she reluctantly told him of his daughter's death. Another neighbor was asked to go outside to make an official identification of the body. While he did that, his wife sat in the house and remembered the last times she'd seen Martha alive, the previous Saturday night at the Moxley home and at the high school the previous week. So alive and so vibrant. Then, when her husband returned grim, the two decided he should go over to Greenwich High School, to football practice, in order to notify Martha's brother, John, and bring him home. A phone call to the football coach had already brought news of the tragedy, and, without telling John why, the coach had sent his player home. Meanwhile, the neighbor had returned from the high school locker room, and he approached John in front of his home as he was about to enter the front door. The neighbor then broke the news about Martha's murder to John, and the distraught teenager's only response was to throw a punch at the man. Trying to console him, the neighbor held out his arms to prevent John from going into the living room, where Dorthy was sitting in a state of shock. John brushed by the man, saying "That's my sister," and the mother and son then engaged in a long, sorrowful embrace. When John finally looked past his mother to the Moxley family grounds, the scene outside that greeted him must have seemed straight out of hell.[13]

Numbers of uniformed and plainclothes officers looking for evidence walked across the lawn around the pine tree where Martha's body lay. Her head was covered with so much blood that one of the officers thought Martha was a redhead. In randomly walking over the killing ground, stretching upward toward the Skakel home on Otter Rock Drive, they were walking over the very lawn across which the victim's body had been dragged the previous night. Many others, some volunteers and some simply curiosity seekers, walked through this same area. A call was made to the state's chief medical examiner, who was unavailable, since he reported he was dealing with a very heavy caseload. No qualified individual was sent to replace him. By midafternoon, the media had gotten word of the murder, and they began to arrive. Most acted responsibly. But there were others. One reporter saw Michael Skakel and another teenaged boy talking. She approached Michael and, microphone in hand, asked him if it was his mother who had died choking on a piece of steak, mixing up Ann Skakel's cause of death with that of his aunt. The boy broke into uncontrollable sobs and bolted away.

The Greenwich Police Department contacted the state police, and the state police ID unit quickly responded. Detectives from the Greenwich police and the Connecticut State Police searched the Moxley house's yard. On the front lawn, they found, gleaming in the afternoon sun, the broken-off head of a woman's golf club. The six-iron clubhead was from a rare set of golf clubs sponsored by Toney Penna. A while later, higher up on the side lawn and in a large puddle of what appeared to be coagulating blood, an eighteen-inch part of the shaft of a club was discovered. The handle of the golf club was not found, nor will it likely ever be, though decades later two of the first police officers on the scene will insist they saw it protruding from Martha's skull.[14]

The police had begun theorizing on what kind of individual could have done this terrible thing. The nearby Connecticut Turnpike seemed a tantalizing possibility to explain where the murderer came from since it is one of the busiest roadways in America and one that attracts hitchhikers and vagrants from just about anywhere. The investigators seemed to assume that the killer could not have come from the immediate, protected peninsula where they stood. In subsequent weeks, many valuable police hours would be wasted looking for a vagrant who'd happened into Belle Haven and they assumed had wantonly struck down this innocent child. This police preoccupation with the outsider-vagrant theory flew in the face of another very glaring discovery made the very first day. An almost-complete set of women's Toney Penna golf clubs was found in the Skakel household that first afternoon, a set of clubs that was missing its six iron. The handles of all of the clubs discovered in the house that day bore the name Ann Reynolds, the late Mrs. Skakel's maiden name.

The Greenwich police did not entirely rule out those close at hand in the first days of this investigation. Their cursory search of the Skakel home that Julie Skakel verbally agreed to as well as the questioning of her and her brothers, Tom and Michael, bore this out. Then there was the burly looking man that special police officer Anthony Whelan had observed on two occasions the night before. A neighbor fit this description, and police questioned this twenty-six-year-old, but found that he had an airtight alibi for the evening, since he'd been at a friend's house in Old Greenwich watching *The French Connection.* More ominously, some of the Belle Haven residents looked nervously down Walsh Lane, toward the home of what they considered a strange person, a twenty-six-year-old heavy-drinking Yale graduate and army veteran. The preceding April, Raymond Todd Becker,* a good-looking, tall young man, had been discovered by one woman trying to force his way through her first-floor French doors and into the living room. When confronted, Raymond, who was recently a graduate student in the business school at Columbia University, had darted off without explanation. Early the next morning, an apologetic Raymond had showed up at this neighbor's front door to explain that all he'd wanted to do was to look at the neighbor's family dog. Hearing this background on Becker, the police immediately went to his house, where, since his father's death two years earlier, he'd lived alone with his mother. Neighbors felt his drinking was somewhat related to his grieving over his dad's death.

At the Beckers' home, detectives discovered that Raymond owned a cache of girly magazines and was prone to masturbate into condoms, which he then saved. Police, given an informal signed permission by Mrs. Becker, searched the home and found, among other items, a box of contraceptives and a bloodstained shirt. The electrified detectives now read Raymond Todd Becker his rights. Later that afternoon, he and his mother were taken down to police headquarters, where Becker was interviewed. Mrs. Becker had gone down to the Belle Haven Club for dinner on the previous night, but Becker had stayed at home. Like Bruce Atwell, another future suspect in the case, Becker had sat by himself watching the movie *The French Connection.* Not much of an alibi. Police took a sample lock of his hair. Raymond Becker remained a prime suspect for some time, even though he passed a second polygraph test that the police gave him. The first test had proven inconclusive, possibly a result of the medication Becker was taking to curb his attraction to alcohol. Becker was finally excluded as a suspect when blood tests showed that the bloodstains on his shirt were, in fact, his own blood that he'd shed during a nosebleed.

During the waning hours on Halloween day, the police investigation found evidence that the location where the body was found was not where Martha Moxley had been murdered. Detectives followed a blood trail they'd found under the pine tree, up along a path, one that stretched across the Moxley driveway. Investigators determined that the fatal first blows were struck where they'd found the pool of coagulating blood, a location 150 feet closer to the Skakel property, and that the victim, face down, had been dragged to her final resting place under the pine, probably to hide the body.[15] (Much later, in 1993, a special task force conducted an in-depth analysis and reconstruction of the crime scene. Because of this, we were able to learn much more about the case's facts. These findings will be discussed later.)

In his 1998 book, *Murder in Greenwich: Who Killed Martha Moxley?* former Los Angeles detective Mark Fuhrman refers to what he considers the continuing negligence by Connecticut's chief medical examiner's office and its failure to establish a time of death.[16] Determining the time of death is never simple. This is an area of forensic pathology. (There is an in-depth discussion of this issue in my earlier book, *Cracking Cases*.) Dr. Elliot Gross, the chief medical examiner, arrived in Greenwich early on Saturday, November 1, and he walked the crime scene—though, with the body already removed, his finding anything there was highly improbable. He also was shown an eight-millimeter movie of the crime scene and studied black-and-white photos taken there the day before. Since these photos were not in color, no real determination on the effects of lividity on the body could be made. Because of this late start on the case, the best Dr. Gross could do was to estimate the time of death between 9:30 PM on Thursday and 5:00 AM on Friday, a finding he announced to the media. This estimate was substantially based on the corpse's having started to come out of rigor mortis. On that Saturday, Dr. Gross performed a lengthy, six-hour-and-five-minute autopsy on the victim's body. Toxicology reports would later indicate that Martha Moxley was not under the influence of alcohol or drugs at the time of her death.[17]

These negative toxicology reports were important since this indicated that her judgment was not impaired when she was attacked. The full autopsy report has never been made public, though highlights of it were announced upon its completion that Saturday evening by the chief state medical examiner. At least four severe blows to the head with a blunt instrument were the principal cause of Martha's death. At least one of the blows caused a severe fracture of her skull, the wound through which the family physician had been able to see into the victim's cerebral cavity. The head of the golf club, presumably swung with great force, appeared to be the murder weapon. There was a three-inch impression on the left, downward side of the victim's face. This would later be attributed by the medical examiner to the victim's face lying on the murder weapon's shaft. In addition to the blows to the head, the attacker had stabbed the victim through her neck with the broken shaft of the golf club, severing her windpipe, but not cutting any arteries. This occurred with such force that strands of hair from her head had been forced all the way through her neck. This stabbing was done in a right-to-left motion.[18]

Suffice it to say that Martha Moxley's murder was obviously committed with great passion. The savageness of the attack was self-evident. And even though the victim's jeans and underpants had been pulled down and scratch marks were found on her thighs, possibly from the assailant's fingernails, there was no further evidence of a sexual assault. Even though the majority of the detectives and policemen at the crime scene had no experience investigating a brutal homicide such as this one, this conclusion should have been most obvious. Would a total stranger, such as a vagrant passing through that secluded section of Greenwich that night, likely commit such a crime? Possibly a psychotic, but that was not at all probable. The murderer was someone full of rage and an individual who, in all probability, knew Martha Moxley. So much for the early theory that Belle Haven's proximity to the Connecticut Turnpike and its constant flow of outsiders could have provided the pool of suspects for this killing. Yet Greenwich police received hundreds of tips on turnpike vagrants, all in response to teletypes the police kept sending out for weeks after the murder.

As the Greenwich police questioned the Skakel family, certain hard facts emerged. Tommy was established as the last person to see Martha before the murderous attack. Michael described his getting into the Skakel family Lincoln with Martha and two other girls at about 9:30 PM. A few minutes later, Tommy came down to the car, purportedly looking for one of his music tapes, and then got into the front seat, right next to Martha. From the backseat, Michael said he saw his brother try to place his hand on Martha's thigh—several times—moves she brushed away. Tommy said that he did no such thing. At about 9:25, Rushton Jr., nineteen, who was home for a long weekend from Dartmouth College where he was a sophomore, came out to the car with his younger brother, John, age sixteen, and their cousin Jim Terrien. The three of them needed the Lincoln to take Jimmy back to his house, called Sursum Corda, about ten miles and twenty minutes away in backcountry Greenwich. The kids already in the car then all had to get out. Michael then opted to make the trip and said he asked Martha if she wanted to come along and that she declined the invitation. The four teenagers departed in the Lincoln, and, after watching parts of a *Monty Python* show on television, they purportedly did not return to Belle Haven until 11:30 PM, nearly two hours later.

The next day, Tommy Skakel got home from his school's football practice after dark, at 5:30 PM. This was when police questioned him and took him downtown, where he made a formal statement. Tom was the last person seen with Martha, as established by his sister Julie, after the two had gotten out of the Lincoln. In his statement, Tom described how Martha and he had talked for a few moments and that she'd headed for home around 9:30. A little while later, a friend of Julie Skakel's showed up at the front door, needing a set of keys to a second family car so Julie could drive her home. Tom looked in on Bruce Atwell and joined the new tutor to watch *The French Connection* in the master bedroom, then went to his room to work on some homework, specifically a paper on Abraham Lincoln, before going to bed around 11:00 PM. Except for the part about his not trying to put his hand on Martha's leg, Tommy's story matched Michael's.[19]

Rushton Skakel returned from his hunting trip on Saturday. Shocked by Martha's murder, he promised to cooperate as fully as possible with the police. The police asked Rushton about his son Steven's reportedly having heard a loud argument under his bedroom window the night of the murder. The police had gotten wind of this from the family of one of the boy's friends with whom he'd ridden the school bus on Friday morning. Rushton promised to ask Steven about this and later reported to police that the boy had actually been awakened by Martha Moxley's laughter and not by a loud fight. Mr. Skakel signed a consent form allowing police to search his premises; it was a form similar to the one signed by the Becker family. This cooperation extended to a search of the ski lodge that Rushton owned in Windham, New York. However, the search of the Skakel home in Belle Haven was unlike the all-out effort made by police at the Becker home. At the Skakel house, investigators performed only a perfunctory walk-through. Garbage pails were not emptied, and there was no check of the clothes washer and dryer. The police did take a companion club from the Toney Penna set, a five iron. All in all, the Skakel family, led by Rushton, seemed to be as cooperative as possible, and they even promised to conduct their own search, too.

On the following Friday, November 7, with Rushton Skakel's consent, Tommy and his father were taken to the Connecticut State Police Troop I barracks in Bethany, where the son was given a polygraph test at the forensic laboratory. The results of the three individual tests administered were inconclusive. This was attributed to Tom's being so exhausted and nervous. Two days later, again at the Bethany facilities, Tom took another test, and this time he passed. This did not mean, however, that Tom was no longer a suspect. Neighborhood children had come forward and reported that they'd seen Tommy and Martha engaging in some flirtatious, pushing-shoving horseplay around 9:30 on that Thursday evening, after the Lincoln had left. On Wednesday, December 13, police again asked

Tom to come in, and they reinterviewed him. After getting the teenager's permission, they also took several strands of his hair.

As rumors began to swirl through Greenwich, the police chief and the local paper asked for public restraint and impartiality. At his private school, Tom was already known for his hot-tempered ways by both faculty and fellow students. It did not help his situation that it turned out that the paper on Lincoln he'd said he had been working on that night was on a different topic, for a class in anthropology. As the weeks rolled on, Tom's behaviors increasingly became the subject of public scrutiny and gossip. Stories emerged from his school and other sources about his extremely violent outbursts, such as his nearly strangling to death a fellow student for a perceived slight and his ripping a door off of its hinges another time. People following the case increasingly heard rumors about a cover-up and how the family fortune and the "Kennedy connection" were behind it. Finally, the following January, Rushton Skakel's cooperation with the police ended, and he dug in his heels.

When originally requested, Rushton had agreed to turn over Tom's school records to the police. However, a few days later Mr. Skakel personally served the police with a letter in which he officially withdrew this consent. Within the hour, Rushton and Joseph Donovan, a high-powered Great Lakes Carbon attorney, dropped in at a neighbor's home in Belle Haven. While waiting to be served refreshments, Rushton suffered chest pains, and an ambulance soon rushed him to Greenwich Hospital. Police arrived at the Belle Haven residence and were told by Donovan that Rushton had related that he'd had a meeting at the boys' private school earlier that day. He also mentioned that Rushton had further explained that he'd just received a phone call and had gotten some bad news. The police then went to the hospital and attempted to interview Mr. Skakel there, but they were told by a Catholic priest, a family friend, that they could have only a few minutes with him. Rushton brought this conversation to a quick end by referring the police to Emmanuel Margolis, a prominent Stamford defense counsel who would go on to represent all of the Skakel family and their household staff, including the tutor, Bruce Atwell.[20]

During most of the year that followed, Tom Skakel remained the only prime suspect in the case. Tommy was absent from school for long periods of time and then was hospitalized for bleeding ulcers, a condition often related to alcohol or drug abuse. In late March, Donald A. Browne, the Fairfield County state's attorney, now confronted with a very experienced and seasoned defense lawyer and no further police access to any of the Skakel family members, publicly stated that the investigation was being impeded by the lack of cooperation of a particular family. Residents of Belle Haven and all of Greenwich did not have to stretch their imaginations very far to surmise the identity of that family and that Tommy Skakel was still the prime suspect. For a few weeks, Tom traveled to Ireland to stay with his aunt. Even this trip set off rumors that he'd fled the country. There was talk at this time, much of it originating with Rushton Skakel, that Tommy had undergone a series of tests and that their results indicated that he was neither the murderer of Martha Moxley nor was capable of such a crime. In telling the Moxley family about these tests, Rushton had said that his attorney had advised against his sharing the test results with the police or anyone else. Shortly thereafter, the Moxley family retained their own counsel to assist them in seeing that the killer of their daughter was brought to justice.

The spotlight of police suspicion lingered on Tom Skakel during the first nine months of 1976, though their interest in him began to wane. Perhaps it's because of the battery of tests that Rushton Skakel had talked about, even though the Moxley family's attorney, let alone the police, were never shown these test results. From the very start of the investigation, police had to track down scores of potential leads, such as a sex offender who lived in the Bronx and was home with his wife the night of the murder. On another tip, the New Rochelle police were told of a sex offender who habitually kept golf clubs in his car. In the last year, however, the clubs had been kept in a locker in a country club in Westchester County. Soon after the murder, there was an anonymous letter to the Moxley household from New York, written in a sort of broken English, warning police to scrutinize the "demoralized, rotten boys" who lived in their vicinity. The list of vague, time-consuming, and unproductive leads went on and on. This legwork was against the backdrop of police preoccupation with the hundreds of vagrants they'd heard about and, first and foremost, Raymond Todd Becker, and then Tommy Skakel.[21]

A few weeks after the murder, two Greenwich police detectives went to the private school where the Skakels' tutor, Bruce Atwell, taught and was an assistant football coach. In college, Atwell's football prowess had been so recognized that there was even a credible rumor that he might be drafted by a team in the National Football League. This was in spite of his playing at Williams College, a very small school, but one with an outstanding reputation for academics and a very selective admissions policy. The two detectives approached Atwell during football practice and watched in amazement as Atwell mouthed off at them, claiming he wasn't going to give them a thing that could be used against Tommy Skakel. They quickly left, but the performance had made a deep impression on them. Was the tutor/coach overreacting to impress the Skakel family? Was he a little deranged? Or did this display serve to throw even more light onto Tom Skakel and, thus, away from himself? Later on, one of the Moxley neighbors, the mother of one of Martha's friends, suggested that Mr. Atwell be considered as a suspect. She told police that he regularly sunbathed, completely nude, in the gazebo on the Skakel grounds. Moreover, police knew that Atwell had not been able to pass a polygraph test, though he did not outright fail that exam. Much later he would fail a second lie detector test. Finally, there was the question of whether the Skakel family was actively setting up Bruce Atwell as a prime suspect. Shortly after the murder, Rushton Skakel and his seven children, along with Jimmy Terrien, retired to the family ski lodge in Windham, New York, for a long weekend of talk. Bruce Atwell was invited to join them for the family discussion, but he had to drive up later on, with two of the Skakel boys. He left after only one day. Shortly thereafter, Rusthon Skakel began to express displeasure with Bruce Atwell.

Then, almost a year after the murder, the Greenwich police remembered the football practice incident when word trickled down to them that Bruce Atwell had been arrested on Nantucket Island for burglary and felony theft by police a few months earlier, in the summer of 1976. Checking further, detectives found that, according to police and many witnesses, Atwell's behavior had become very bizarre. He'd worked all that summer as a bouncer in an island club that catered to a very young and attractive crowd. Perhaps to impress the ladies, Atwell took to positioning himself at the door in a three-piece white suit, his shirt open down his chest, with shiny white shoes. He drank heavily and seemed to do everything possible to make himself conspicuous, such as habitually combing his long hair with a large black comb. After his night's work was completed, Atwell would drink and cavort around on the dance floor and, later on, go to another, smaller bar, where he would continue to drink. Finally, on his way to the house he'd rented, Atwell would stagger onto people's front lawns and steal the ornaments and other loose objects he'd find there. He even broke into several homes and a boat. He liked to bury his loot. Atwell eventually tried to sell some of what he'd stolen, but he picked a police informant as his fence. Tipped off, the Nantucket police finally raided his home and dug up or otherwise found $4,000 worth of stolen artifacts and property. Atwell was arrested and charged with burglary and grand larceny, the latter a felony. After all was said and done, he eventually got probation and served no time.

Realistically or not, all of this put Atwell at the very top of the Greenwich police's new list of murder suspects.[22] In retrospect, there are a few salient points that jump out, even twenty-seven years later, that argue against the possibility that he killed Martha Moxley. Bruce Atwell reported for work the very afternoon of the murder. Unless he was a psychotic, is it feasible that a new family tutor would look across the two hundred yards separating his own new domicile and the Moxley home and instantly determine that he was going to club to death the pretty, teenaged blond girl across the way? And did he even glimpse Martha that first afternoon, before supposedly bludgeoning her to death? And with a golf club he'd conveniently found in the Skakel backyard?

Suffice it to say for now that it is not at all logical that members

of the Skakel family would indulge in cover-up behavior to excul-
pate their brand-new employee and houseguest, especially when
this activity would inevitably shorten by one the short list of suspects, thus even more closely casting the investigative net toward
one of their own two sons. Certainly, Bruce Atwell himself could not
have conducted the actions necessary for a cover-up without
drawing attention to himself. His getting caught disposing of any
forensic evidence would have led to his immediate arrest. But, as
they already had with the Connecticut Turnpike vagrants and with
Thomas Skakel, the police again had no forensic evidence to link
him to the crime.

In the next few years, investigators tried diligently to build a case
against Bruce Atwell. They even attempted to have his ex-wife lure
him into self-incriminating statements, having electronic eavesdrop-
ping devices recording their every word. The new prime suspect himself, however, did nothing to cool things down. Instead, his continuing erratic behaviors over the next twenty-two years simply served
to fire up investigative interest in him. Atwell went on to be arrested
on a number of occasions, but only once for assault and battery. He
was institutionalized for his alcohol abuse and mental problems.
Even more than the fruitless search for Martha Moxley's turnpike
killer, the Atwell imbroglio served to distract investigators from pursuing leads that were far more promising.

The Martha Moxley murder case began to recede into the background. There were the usual news accounts about the killing on the
first anniversary of the murder. Occasionally, the national media
would decide to revisit this notorious, unsolved crime, invariably
mentioning the tragedy's connection to the Kennedys. For the
Greenwich police, Tom Skakel seemed to fade from the radar as a
top suspect, replaced by Bruce Atwell, who made a convenient reference point whenever journalists asked authorities about where the
case was going. In the fall of 1976, Rushton Skakel finally termi-
nated Atwell, for no apparent reason, even refusing to pay him back
wages until a mutual friend intervened. Atwell was then off on his
own odyssey. His academic career in ruins over the suspicion cast on
him, he drifted into the commodities field and moved south, to

Florida. There, he ran into more bad fortune. The brokerage firm that Atwell joined was subsequently prosecuted for fraud and theft and closed down. Later on, Atwell's parents went on to say that their son's being hounded by the police and the media had intensified what they recognized as his severe mental problems. Eventually, their son moved to Canada with a girl he'd met in Florida and got married. A few years later, the couple divorced. All of that aside, as the years since Mischief Night in 1975 rolled on, even the national media seemed to lose interest in the case.[23]

In 1977 David and Dorthy Moxley moved to New York City. Their remaining child, John, graduated from Greenwich High that year, but the young man felt that he needed another year at the secondary level to regain his senses, so he did his fifth year at Choate, the exclusive prep school in Wallingford, Connecticut, before going on to Ohio Wesleyan for college. David Moxley, putting in his usual grueling schedule, became the national managing partner for Touche, Ross and then was promoted to the top job for the firm's worldwide operations. With the help of his friends at his firm, David was able to prod the Greenwich police into accepting assistance in solving his daughter's murder from the nationally renowned forensic pathologist Dr. Werner Spitz of Detroit (a jurisdiction that for years had the country's highest murder rate) and from other detectives. Dorthy Moxley had to content herself to letting her husband handle the details in pursuing the investigation. Recognizing finally that his strenuous schedule at Touche, Ross had been taking a heavy toll, Mr. Moxley retired from the firm and instead became the managing partner for a firm of high-powered Manhattan attorneys. In 1986 Dorthy Moxley was left to close out the couple's Manhattan apartment and move to the serenity of Annapolis, Maryland, where her husband and she had purchased a waterfront condo to live in during their retirement.

Then, the day before Thanksgiving in 1988, Dorthy returned to New York to find David still in bed late in the morning, dead of a heart attack. He was only fifty-seven. His premature death was hastened, no doubt, by a combination of his grueling work schedule and the anxiety and sadness over Martha's murder, a tragedy that likely haunted him every day of his life.

After David's death, Dorthy moved to Chatham, New Jersey, and then finally to California. Intelligent, poised, and still grief-stricken, Dorthy Moxley decided to pick up where her late husband's efforts had left off and to pursue, with all of her considerable intellect and vigor, the investigation into Martha's murder. For starters, she resolved to speak to any and all journalists and investigators who purported to share some of her insatiable interest in finding the murderer. One of these writers would prove a particularly worthwhile investment of Mrs. Moxley's time and energy.[24]

Not all of America's journalists had forgotten about the Moxley murder. Leonard Levitt was a former *Time* magazine star writer who had, for one reason or another, left that publication to become a freelance journalist. My coauthor, Tom O'Neil, a former editor of *Newark!* magazine, remembers Levitt from his 1969–1970 reporting for *Time* on the wholesale indictments of Newark mayor Hugh Addonizio, three officials from his cabinet, and three members of the city council, all on dozens of counts of municipal corruption. Levitt practically lived in Newark and led much of the national coverage of this municipal crime story. Suffice it to say, Levitt would prove to be just the journalistic bulldog that the Moxley case so desperately needed.

One of the first discoveries Len Levitt made in his work on the Moxley case was that there was very little to discover in the police records. This came through to him during the course of a lengthy interview with Dorthy Moxley. The Greenwich police had put very little on the official record. Also, as we have previously noted, the state's medical examiner would not allow reporters access to his autopsy. Dr. Gross also refused anyone access to the color photos he had taken that Saturday after the murder, claiming these were his personal property. Incensed, in 1983 Levitt joined forces with *Greenwich Time,* the community's daily newspaper, and went to the Connecticut Freedom of Information Agency and sued for the release of these records. Levitt and company would win the battle but, regrettably, not the war. Greenwich police then went to court to obtain the unprecedented right to edit Levitt's eventual story, a suit that they lost. No matter. The police had already redacted large portions of the record and other important information that didn't have to be inked over, since it was never recorded in the first place. For instance, there was no mention of Michael Skakel's saying he'd seen his brother, Tom, running his hand up and down Martha's thigh while they sat in the family Lincoln and her rejecting his advances. Then, after all Levitt did, both *Greenwich Time* and its sister publication, the *Stamford Advocate*, refused to print Levitt's eye-opening story.[25]

In April of 1991, in Palm Beach, Florida, rape charges were filed against William Kennedy Smith, a nephew of the late president John F. Kennedy and a cousin of the Skakel family. Ironically, this case served to reawaken public interest in and, hence, journalistic coverage of the Martha Moxley murder. The Kennedy family retained a top defense attorney, Roy Black, to defend Willie Smith. Contacted by the defense team, I worked on this case and eventually testified in court. I've used the word *ironically* here since, though Willie Smith was acquitted of all charges, the media began again to focus its attention on the troubles of the Kennedy family and also, by extension, its cousins through marriage, the Skakel family. And a great deal of this media excitement was fanned by a newer genre, the so-called tabloid television programs. One such tabloid TV report served to generate three more, and so on. Succumbing to the gathering storm of public interest, on June 21, 1991, *Greenwich Time* and the *Stamford Advocate* finally published Len Levitt's story on the Moxley case and its botched investigation. The Associated Press immediately picked up on Levitt's meticulous work, and his findings appeared in hundreds of newspapers around the nation. Dorthy Moxley and her son, John, now stepped forward and announced that they would more than double the standard $20,000 for information leading to a conviction, making the sum $50,000. Additionally, the Moxley family would fund an 800-number tip line. The Moxleys made this announcement on August 9, 1991. At that time, Donald Browne, the Bridgeport and Fairfield County state's attorney, the Greenwich police chief, and the state police announced that the case was formally being reinvestigated, using any and all state resources deemed necessary.[26] These resources included the Connecticut State Police Forensic Laboratory in Meriden, where I was the director and the state's chief criminalist. A special office in the Greenwich Police Department would be established, and that's where calls on the new hotline would be received.

The following year, Rushton Skakel quietly met with James Murphy, head of Sutton Associates, a detective agency based on Long Island. Murphy, a former veteran FBI agent, was instructed by Mr. Skakel to dig into the facts, such as those that could be established, and to pull no punches on what he and his associates at Sutton were able to find. These findings were to be totally confidential. Rushton Skakel was very clear on what he wanted done, and he was willing to pay a large sum of money to determine if someone other than a member of his family had committed the crime. Or, if Sutton found that the murderer was a Skakel, the agency was to help the family establish as good a defense as possible. Pertaining to the confidentiality requirement, all of the Sutton investigators would have to sign an oath promising this secrecy.[27]

In 1993 the media surge continued. Author Dominick Dunne met with Dorthy Moxley. Dunne's passion for the case was undoubtedly fired in large part by the fact that his own daughter, Dominique, was murdered, and her assailant went to prison for only two and a half years. Dunne wove many of the facts and rumors on the Moxley case into a novel, *A Season in Purgatory*, a best-seller that later was produced as a made-for-television movie. More Americans now began taking an interest in the unsolved Martha Moxley case. Media and general public interest, though, are no substitute for hard evidence.[28]

In October of 1993, after an exhaustive analysis, I authored a voluminous review of the available evidence, forensic and investigative, a document based on the autopsy and all of the nonredacted police reports. This report included a reconstruction of the crime and how it took place at the crime scenes. Its contents were not made public, though, and the following January I announced that, after eighteen months of work, the Connecticut State Forensic Laboratory had done all it could to solve the crime. I put out that statement partially because reporters and others hounded us on a regular basis. The media wanted news of a dramatic breakthrough in this investigation.

There is an old football coach's saying about how a particular team will do: you cannot make chicken salad if you have no chicken. The report, as copious as it was, was based only on the evidence we had been given, data that was then nearly twenty years old.

The media attention that had been gathering steam in the early part of the 1990s did not all serve to unravel the Gordian knot that was tied around and throughout the Moxley case. In 1991 an unofficial source told a reporter from the tabloid program *Hard Copy* that Martha Moxley had been stabbed four times. This was not true, and anyone with any real familiarity with the facts of the case should have known better. Then, in 1993, cameras from the tabloid show *A Current Affair* tracked down Bruce Atwell as he sat sipping a soft drink in Boston's fashionable Fanueil Hall marketplace, badgering the obviously upset former tutor on what he knew about the murder. Atwell did add one element to his account, that he'd heard someone or something moving in the bushes when he'd come downstairs at the maid's request. He'd looked about, had seen nothing, and had returned upstairs to his movie watching in the master bedroom. Hearing this, Greenwich police scoffed and pointed to the statement as one more erratic act by Mr. Atwell, who was still very much their prime suspect. Each passing month seemed to bring another media excess, many times from the original supermarket tabloids. Two strands of hair found at the murder scene provided cannon fodder for some of this misinformation. Upon reexamination of Martha Moxley's clothing, a single fragment of Caucasian hair, too small to provide any DNA evidence, was found on the victim's jeans. She had been sitting in the front seat of the Skakel family car that evening, next to Tom Skakel, and with two other teenaged boys in the backseat. My laboratory had determined this fragment of hair to be of human and Caucasian origin. This strand could have come from any of those three boys. A second strand of Negroid hair was discovered at the crime scene. One of the Greenwich police officers was African American, and he was, in all probability, the source of this strand of hair. Yet these minor facts generated more than their fair share of tabloid reaction.

Responsible journalists, however, were providing accurate and hard-hitting stories on the case. On November 3, 1995, Dorthy Moxley convened a dinner at the Belle Haven Club for all the task force investigators who had worked diligently for months on solving her daughter's murder. I was also invited. This was the first time I had ever met Mrs. Dorthy Moxley and her son, John. Their combined sincerity and deep, passionate love for Martha touched me deeply. During the evening's conversation, many questions were put to me by those present about the recently adjudicated O. J. Simpson case. Tim Dumas was also in attendance, and, in his fine book, he later described the somber feeling that permeated the room during the occasion marking the twentieth anniversary of this awful and unsolved crime.[29] Dumas also described the excitement that the journalists shared with one another in anticipation of a story that Len Levitt had been working on for quite some time.

Now a reporter with *Newsday*, the large and influential Long Island newspaper, Levitt was getting close to breaking his story. A little more than three weeks later, on November 26, Levitt dropped his bombshell. Based on leaks from the Sutton agency, the Skakel family's detectives, Levitt authored a story about how Tommy Skakel had changed his account of what had happened on the night of October 30–31, 1975.[30] Tom, instead of going to his bedroom to do some homework, now admitted that he'd gone back outside for a prearranged date with Martha Moxley, and the two had engaged in some heavy adolescent petting, each of them achieving orgasm. Following this, Tommy had gone back to his bedroom and to sleep. This interlude concluded, according to Tom, about 9:50 PM. This was all in spite of Tom's eventually passing a lie detector test in 1976, when, in response to a question about the last time he had seen Martha Moxley, he had lied and said it was twenty minutes earlier.[31]

In the first week of December, Levitt followed up that huge story with one about Michael Skakel. The younger brother now also had admittedly lied to the police and subsequently claimed that, after he and his two older brothers had returned from their visit to the Terrien household at about 11:30 PM, he had gone back out into the night. Intoxicated and probably stoned, Michael had wandered about the Belle Haven neighborhood, peeking into windows, including one that he hoped was Martha Moxley's bedroom. Later on, Michael would expand on this story, due, very possibly, to his hearing about a report from the news media that we had found DNA evidence at the crime scene. Michael then added the fact that he had even climbed a tree behind Martha's house so he could throw pebbles at her window and otherwise attempt to get her attention. When Martha failed to appear, Michael reported that he engaged in masturbation until he had an orgasm.

These two news stories created a firestorm of media and public reaction. And, for the very first time since the murder itself, Michael Skakel became a suspect in the eyes of the investigative team.[32] This seems somewhat hard to believe, in hindsight. But poorly conducted investigations have their own unique domino effect. There was no real forensic and pathological analysis at the crime scene on the afternoon of October 31, 1975. These lapses were a prime cause in the investigation's failure to establish the victim's time of death at or about 9:30 to 10:00 PM. Furthermore, the delay in the victim's autopsy proved another primary cause for the guesswork that went into establishing Martha Moxley's time of death. Loud voices and barking dogs were the principal evidence. Michael Skakel had a credible alibi for that time span. Unlike his brother, Tom, he wasn't even given a polygraph test. Michael had been, nearly from the first, almost entirely below the police investigators' radar systems.

Should he have been left off a list of prime suspects? Michael's behaviors were such that several neighbors in Belle Haven who knew both boys well said, in the months immediately following the crime, that Michael was the one quite capable of so violent a crime and that Tom was not. As the months and years dragged on, though, Michael's behaviors began to draw increasing attention. In the very early hours of March 5, 1978, with a date riding in the front passenger seat, Michael drove the Skakel family Jeep on a darkened road through a police barricade at an accident scene in Windham, New York. He was chased and finally caught, after he drove the Jeep into a telephone poll, destroying the vehicle—though, luckily for Michael, neither he nor his girlfriend were harmed. A Skakel family attorney was summoned, and Michael was convicted of all the charges except for driving while under the influence of alcohol. The court made a deal suspending a jail sentence, on the condition that he immediately enter an upscale treatment center in Maine, called Elan. Once there, Michael reportedly tried to escape from this facility three times, and on two occasions he got as far as Boston and New York before being captured and returned.

Not all of the news-program television coverage of the Moxley case has been counterproductive. In early 1996, a man who had also been receiving treatment at the Elan School in Maine at the time Michael Skakel had been a patient there called the tipline of the television show *Unsolved Mysteries*. While he was in group therapy, this fellow patient and others heard Michael Skakel confess to Martha Moxley's murder. Others at Elan reported the same thing had occurred on other occasions, though in each instance Michael later recanted. After two years, Rushton Skakel Sr. took Michael out of Elan and sent his troubled son to other similar institutions, moves that Michael bitterly opposed. Rehabilitation institutions cannot divulge their patient lists to the police or to the media. Backed by his enormous family fortune, Mr. Skakel continued to shuttle Michael to clinics and rehab centers throughout New England, even sending him back to Elan in Maine. This went on for more than a decade, and Michael finally emerged from this treatment cycle in the early nineties. He then earned a bachelor's degree from Curry College in the Boston area, fell in love with a girl who worked as a golf pro, and got married. After having one child, a daughter, the couple eventually divorced. Michael went to work for an environmental company headed by his cousin, Michael Kennedy, but this relationship ended when he became too friendly with the teenaged babysitter with whom the Kennedy cousin had been sleeping. The two parted company, and Michael Skakel later went into commercial real estate, though this endeavor also did not work out. By the time the news of his confessions at the Elan school erupted, Michael Skakel had put on a great deal of excess weight, and the news cameras that now began to seek him out presented the image of an arrogant, bejowled man in his late thirties, his round face set under thinning blond hair. Aside from Bruce Atwell, whom the investigators still considered a suspect, the spotlight of suspicion now glared down on Michael Skakel.[33]

State's Attorney Donald Browne had been increasingly criticized in the media and by Moxley case insiders for not taking the step of convening a one-man grand jury, a Connecticut replacement of the probable cause hearing. Chaired by a sitting judge in total secrecy, this body could then subpoena witnesses and documents. The Sutton Agency's investigators could, for instance, be forced to open up and provide this forum with all their data, no matter what confidentiality agreements the agency had with the Skakel family. In September of 1997, Donald Browne was due to retire. However, Browne announced that he would stay on the job to pursue one case, the unsolved Moxley murder. This development startled many and satisfied few. More time dragged on, and there still did not seem to be any further progress in bringing this murder to trial, in spite of the Sutton disclosures and Michael Skakel's reported confessions.

Things heated up even more when Len Levitt reported on September 30 that Dominick Dunne had possession of the Sutton agency's full reports. As more and more information from the Sutton reports leaked out, observers were amazed to discover that Sutton investigators disclosed that Martha Moxley had suffered a broken nose on the night of her murder. This was news to many, but what really startled the reporters and writers was that Sutton's people could have had access to the full autopsy reports, which had been so carefully guarded. Money, it was being said, could seem to buy most anything. Whether true or not, money could not assure accurate information. Years after Martha Moxley's body was first discovered, the two juvenile officers who were the first police on the scene reported that they each now remembered seeing the still-missing handle of a golf club protruding from the victim's head. Yet neither one had reported this fact in October of 1975. More confusion emerged when false accusations were made that someone had paid the police to conveniently lose this telltale piece of evidence.[34] Along with alleged statements by Ethel Skakel Kennedy that the use of her late husband's family name had to be minimized,[35] these kinds of phony developments only served to drive the tabloid coverage of the case.

Early in 1998, Donald Browne resigned from the state's attorney's office, after years of excellent public service, turning all his cases over to Jonathan Benedict, a thin, poised, and very hard-working prosecutor. He combined a quiet intensity with a great aptitude for scientific and physical evidence. Jonathan for many years has also been a good friend of mine, and we have worked on many homicide cases together. At one point in a murder investigation, Jonathan called me for a last-minute meeting, on the Sunday before the trial. My wife, Margaret, made a Chinese dinner of pressed duck, with all the trimmings, and Jonathan baked a fresh pie. We spent the entire evening discussing the case and the forensic evidence. His passion and devotion to his duties have always impressed me. Thus, I knew, from the moment I heard that he had taken over the Martha Moxley investigation, that this long-unsolved murder stood a good chance of being brought to a conclusion. So it came as no surprise to me that Benedict announced that the Moxley case was going to apply for an eighteen-month, investigative, one-man grand jury. A three-judge panel sitting in New Haven quickly granted Benedict's request.

Judge Aaron Ment, the state bench's chief administrator, chose Judge George N. Thim, age fifty-five, of Trumbull, Connecticut, to be the one-man grand jury. Judge Thim had an excellent reputation, though most of his judicial career had been devoted to civil rather than criminal cases. Earlier in his career, I'd had the pleasure to meet him and work with him on several cases. Judge Thim's grand jury was also charged to formally review the Greenwich Police Department's handling of the case. Michael Skakel was the primary target for this grand jury, though Bruce Atwell and Tom Skakel would also be called as witnesses. Benedict's office was pushing for a felony murder indictment, since whoever killed Martha Moxley, the autopsy showed, had later returned to stab his victim through the neck with the shaft of the golf club, indicating time for premeditation. This was an important factor since there is no longer a Connecticut statute of limitations for the crime of murder. Former Los Angeles Police Department detective Mark Fuhrman laid out much of this material in his book *Murder in Greenwich*.[36] Fuhrman added that the prosecutor's office never considered any kind of a plea bargain in this case.

Judge Thim brought a no-nonsense manner to his proceedings, set in Bridgeport, one that told members of the press that anyone caught attempting to discover anything from inside his proceedings would soon be looking out at the world from a jail cell. Yet the grand jury that was convened in June of 1998 served to draw even more media and public attention to the Moxley case. Dozens of state and national news reporters and photographers swarmed over the steps of the Bridgeport courthouse. This was especially true when Michael Skakel, Thomas Skakel, or Bruce Atwell appeared. I was called to testify later in the summer. Subpoenaed in Florida, where he had moved, Rushton Skakel, now seventy-five, unsuccessfully fought his having to testify before the grand jury due to mental incompetence brought on by progressive dementia. Flanked by his attorney, Richard Lubin, the elder Skakel testified for an hour before Judge Thim on September 9, 1999. Afterward, he spoke to not one of the dozens of journalists who asked him questions.[37]

After taking the full eighteen months allowed by statute, and hearing from more than fifty witnesses, Judge Thim formally concluded his proceedings in December of 1999. His findings were released in January of 2000. Judge Thim wrote, "The evidence shows there is probable cause to support an application for an arrest warrant."[38] Jonathan Benedict then applied to Superior Court Judge Richard F. Cumerford Jr. for an arrest warrant for Michael Skakel, then thirty-nine, for murder, which Judge Cumerford signed on January 18, 2000. Skakel was arrested the next day. Dorthy Moxley and her son, John, expressed their profound relief that they could finally now see that justice would be done over the murder of their beloved Martha. The national news media trumpeted this story. Photos of the Kennedy cousin in handcuffs appeared in papers all over the nation, led by page-one coverage in the regional press. Network newscasts reported the story, complete with footage of Michael flanked by personal bodyguards and his defense lawyer, Michael Sherman of Stratford. Mickey Sherman had a reputation for prodigious work habits, a very sharp approach, and for being very successful in defending particularly controversial clients. Pitted against the much quieter, very well organized Jonathan Benedict, the trial already shaped up to be as intriguing as it was newsworthy.

THE SKAKEL TRIAL

Given the twenty-five-year time span between the commission of the crime and the defendant's ultimately coming before the bar of justice, it's not surprising this trial had important issues to settle before it could begin. The first of these involved the evidence itself. Arguing before Superior Court Judge Maureen Dennis in juvenile court, Mickey Sherman would have to effectively receive from the court a directed verdict of innocence since he would have to show that the case against his client lacked any probable cause. Judges Thim and Cumerford had already found that the evidence more than added up to this standard. And Sherman had another avenue to pursue, arguing that Michael Skakel should be prosecuted as a juvenile because he was fifteen in 1975 when he allegedly killed Martha Moxley. Connecticut law required that a juvenile convicted of murder would have to serve four years in an appropriate institution, one that would emphasize the defendant's rehabilitation. Since Michael Skakel was now thirty-nine, no such facility existed, meaning that any conviction would go unpunished. Jonathan Benedict presented only seven witnesses before Judge Dennis, since the *reasonable* standard he had to meet fell far short of what was required to convict, and he did not want to provide the defense with what would amount to a full-trial dress rehearsal. Benedict's confidence proved well founded, and Judge Dennis ruled that Michael Skakel should be tried as an adult for the 1975 slaying of Martha Moxley.[39] Still, Mickey Sherman appealed Judge Dennis's findings, and these legal motions would have to be resolved prior to a full trial, which meant that the proceedings would be delayed until the spring of 2002. Meanwhile, both sides, the prosecution and the defense, asked me to meet with them. Both Jonathan Benedict and Mickey Sherman asked me about the crime scene reconstruction and the lack of direct physical evidence, such as DNA, semen, or fingerprints, with which to link the accused to the crime.

On Tuesday, May 7, Superior Court Judge John A. Kavenewsky Jr. used his gavel to bring the Skakel trial to order in a packed Norwalk courtroom. Numerous spectators had to be turned away, and an army of television cameras, crews, and reporters stationed themselves under a grove of trees behind the brick one-story courthouse. This array of television equipment and reporters rivaled the media turnout for the O. J. Simpson trial. The courthouse had a gracious ambience, and its graveled apron at the back was soon being called "Pebble Beach North," after the media concentrations on the driveway next to the White House. Dominick Dunne, Leonard Levitt, Timothy Dumas, Mark Fuhrman, and other writers, having labored over this story for years and, in some cases, decades, filed into the courtroom. A half dozen media illustrators were spread around the courtroom. Dorthy and John Moxley sat in the front row, to the left as one looked into the proceedings, while members of the Skakel family were in the same row, to the right, the side closest to the defendant's table. Many of the original police investigators were present, as were prosecutors, lawyers from around the region, and other court observers. Michael Skakel was dressed in a dark blue pin-striped suit and was surrounded by sheriff's deputies whenever he moved anywhere. These were in addition to his own large and muscular bodyguard who accompanied him whenever he ventured out beyond the railing that separated the court from the spectators.

In their opening statements, both sides, predictably, went to the statements Michael Skakel had made over the years, admitting his guilt in the case. "Some people simply cannot keep a secret," Jonathan Benedict said, adding that "as it turns out, he's [Michael Skakel's] been talking about his night of mischief since at least the spring of 1978."After denigrating the alleged statements of admission of guilt by his client when he was at the Elan School, Mickey Sherman argued that the prosecution had "a lot of pieces of a jigsaw puzzle. But the problem is, the jigsaw puzzle pieces don't fit." Sherman cautioned the jury against getting caught up in the emotion of the case and said that the prosecution's evidence amounted to "zilch."

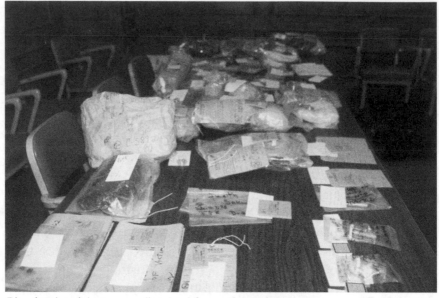

Physical evidence collected from the crime scene and the victim's body.

The prosecution immediately opened its case by calling Dorthy and John Moxley, to the stand and Martha's mother gave the same account she had been relating since 1975. Colleen O'Dwyer provided a very dramatic moment when Mickey Sherman cross-examined her, asking how long it took the girl to run from the pine tree where she found her friend's body to the Moxley home: "Mr. Sherman, it took me a lifetime." Police investigators also were called that first day to establish where the two pieces of the golf club had been found, what they'd discovered indicating where Martha had been initially attacked and subsequently attacked, and the route along which her battered body had been dragged to the pine tree.[40]

The trial's second day was devoted to the physical and forensic evidence. Dr. H. Wayne Carver II, the current state's chief medical examiner, was first called to review the original autopsy performed by Dr. Gross. Carver agreed with the finding that, although the victim's jeans and underwear had been pulled down to her knees, there was no evidence of a sexual assault. He also concluded that, due to the thirty-six hours that elapsed from the finding of Martha Moxley's body until the autopsy, examination of her stomach contents and other tests would prove inconclusive as to the time of her death.

I was called to the stand the same day. Under direct examination I testified that, in my opinion, the victim was first attacked from her left in her family's driveway, where there were a few droplets of blood found on the gravel driveway. The athletic teenager must have then run to her right, across the driveway, and onto her family's lawn. Her attacker, in hot pursuit, would have been carrying the murder weapon, the golf club. Martha Moxley was again attacked approximately 116 feet away from the location of the original assault, at a grassy part of the lawn, where she was killed in "a major assault." The club hit the victim in the head with such ferocity that it broke off and probably flew backward to the left of where the assailant had so savagely struck her. At this point, the perpetrator wielded the sharp-ended club shaft in his hand, and with this he continued to beat his prone victim. He did this with such force that the shaft broke again, and now the assailant held a shard of the golf club's shaft about the size of a long dagger. He used the remaining shaft to stab his victim through her neck so violently that a bundle of hair from her head was pulled entirely through to the other side of her neck, where the shaft's sharp end protruded. Finally, the perpetrator began dragging his victim's body further down the hillside. After approximately eighty feet, he paused and, spotting a large pine tree, pulled her body under its branches. I used charts and diagrams of the area to show the jury and court what my reconstruction showed had occurred. During my testimony I referred to "indirect forensic evidence," a term that Mickey Sherman pointedly decided not to challenge, somewhat sarcastically asking, in effect, "Who would want to take on so well-known a figure as Dr. Lee?" I will address what I meant by this term later in this chapter.

Both Dr. Carver and I testified that there was no physical evidence found from Martha Moxley directly linking her to her assailant. Under cross-examination, I determined that the two hairs taken from a sheet used to cover the body were consistent with hair taken from a brush used by the family tutor, Bruce Atwell. These two specimens were sent out for mitochondrial DNA testing, but there was not a sufficient amount of DNA evidence to precisely individualize Atwell or anyone else. Later in the day, Jonathan Benedict drew laughter when he referred to Michael Skakel's changed story and his alleging that he had masturbated while outside, in a tree, which could later account for any of his DNA being found at the scene. The Skakel family "knew Dr. Lee was entering the investigation," Benedict declared.[41]

The prosecution kept chipping away at Michael Skakel's alibi for the time he allegedly spent riding to the Terrien house that night. Benedict introduced two witnesses, both friends of the Skakel family and one of whom was a dinner guest earlier in the evening when the large group had gone to the Belle Haven Club to eat and drink. This witness, a close friend of Julie Skakel, testified that she saw Michael in his home after the car had left for the Terrien's. Julie didn't drive her home until 9:30 PM. Senior Assistant State's Attorney Susann Gill questioned the friend. "He [Michael] was in the house after the car left?" Answer: "Yes." Question: "Any doubt?" Answer: "No."[42] Later in the trial, the 3:00 AM whereabouts of the cousin, Jimmy Terrien, came into question. Why couldn't his mother, Georgeann Terrien, find him when Dorthy Moxley had woken her up with her frantic call that next morning? Terrien would testify that he'd been having an affair with an older married woman and had slipped out of his house without his mother's knowledge.

The Skakel trial continued on through the month of May. Judge Kavenewsky heard arguments from the defense on why evidence should be introduced that would establish Bruce Atwell, the Skakels' tutor, as the murderer. Judge Kavenewsky did not permit most of what Mickey Sherman wanted to be used. Final arguments were made just prior to the Memorial Day weekend, and the jury of six men and six women began their deliberations on Monday, June 3. Three days passed without any verdict. Then, on Friday, June 7, the jury returned, and the foreman declared that Michael Skakel was guilty of first-degree murder in the death of fifteen-year-old Martha Moxley. Dorthy Moxley and her son, John, triumphantly stood on the steps of the Norwalk courthouse, addressing the media and the world. "This is Martha's day," Mrs. Moxley justly shouted. And,

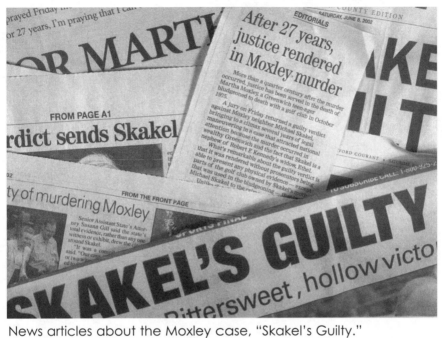

News articles about the Moxley case, "Skakel's Guilty."

though no amount of money or power would ever bring her daughter back, the Moxleys had finally achieved some form of closure over the death of their beloved Martha.

Judge Kavenewsky set Michael Skakel's sentencing for later that summer, August 28 and 29. Again, the media seemed to descend on the Norwalk courthouse. A long line of spectators stood outside the front doors, and many were out back, mingling with the television crews. When the doors swung open, the media and the early-arriving spectators were admitted to the courtroom. The Moxley and Skakel families again sat at opposite ends of the front row, separated at the middle by a single spectator. When Michael Skakel was ushered in, the Skakel family members stood in deference, and, for an instant, it seemed as though others would rise. Dorthy Moxley's quiet voice was heard: "I'm not standing for him." Judge Kavenewsky then heard witnesses for both sides. The next morning, Thursday, August 29, Michael Skakel was sentenced to twenty years to life in prison for his crime. Prior to the sentencing, the defendant took the

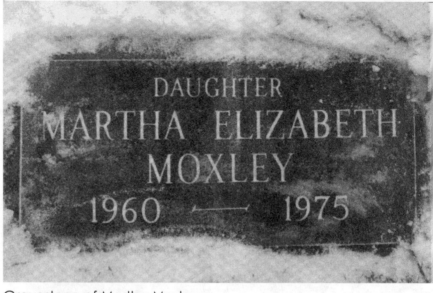

Gravestone of Martha Moxley.

stand and wept. "I didn't do it," he said, the first public statement he had ever uttered on the crime. Dorthy Moxley told reporters outside that she was sympathetic toward her daughter's murderer, though she thought the sentence was fair. "It's my nature to be sympathetic. But he still has to be punished for what he did to Martha." John Moxley remembered the nightmare of learning about his sister's murder while sitting on a bench in his football uniform. "My father was away. I felt I wasn't up to the responsibility of being the man of the house." John also said that his sister's violent death was the one subject his father, David Moxley, could never bring himself to discuss with his son, even up until his premature death. This drama played itself out on Thursday, August 29, 2002, just thirteen days after what should have been Martha Moxley's forty-second birthday.

With its oversights, the Skakel case provides several valuable lessons for the homicide investigator. This may seem a harsh statement, and it is not one that I am making in a glib manner. First and foremost is the need for a prompt autopsy. Many critical facts can be wholly or at least partially determined if an autopsy is completed within three to twelve hours of the victim's death. The time of death is one crucial determination that can be established if the forensic evidence associated with the body is promptly examined. A microscopic examination of stomach contents, against the time of the victim's last meal, if known, is one crucial source of information. If the meal is undigested or only partially digested, then the time of death can be estimated accordingly. Lividity, the skin's becoming discolored due to the settlement of red blood cells in the small blood vessels, is another critical source of information. In the Martha Moxley murder, Dr. Elliott Gross did not start his autopsy until the next noon, almost twenty-four hours after the body was found and an estimated thirty-eight hours after the time of death. This was a contributing factor to this murder's not being solved for so long and for its having so many unanswered questions. In addition, all of the trace evidence on her body, hair, and clothing were not collected and preserved during the autopsy.

During the Skakel case's trial, I used the term "indirect forensic evidence." The lead defense lawyer argued that he did not want to challenge me on the use of this term. I know there is an honored legal adage that holds that counsel should never ask a witness a question unless he knows what answer this query will elicit. In this case, the indirect forensic evidence referred to the case's *missing forensic evidence.* Detectives did not find any bloody clothing inside any of the residences in Belle Haven, especially inside the Skakel household. Yet there must have been considerable blood spatter as a result of the terrible and savage beating inflicted by the murderer on his victim. Where did this all go? Where was the missing handle of the Toney Penna golf club? This was the leather part of the club's shaft that had the Skakel family name (Reynolds) imprinted on it. An instrument like that had to be deliberately removed and taken to a point of disposal. Where was any blood evidence, if any existed, from the murderer? With a beating that furious, one fierce enough to result in a broken golf shaft, very possibly blood will transfer to the suspect's clothing and shoes.

Let me provide you with an example where indirect forensic evidence actually was the key to solving a bloody homicide. Several years ago in a rural section of Connecticut, a housewife purportedly came home from a weekend trip to find her husband dead of a shotgun blast. His body lay in the family's attached garage. I was called to the scene, and, to my astonishment, there was absolutely no evidence of any blood spatter anywhere. Aside from the body, the garage was in pristine condition. I told the police investigators of my surprise, and they quickly began questioning the victim's wife about this. Under this pressure, the wife confessed to her husband's murder and to her having spent the entire weekend cleaning up the mess his killing had left. The absence of evidence is equally as important as the presence of evidence.

In the Skakel case, detectives made the mistake of not properly preserving the crime scenes. True, police had used sawhorses and crime scene tape to rope off what they initially thought was the murder scene. However, these precautions did not hold back the rush of outsiders and the media. Critical and irreplaceable scientific evidence was inevitably trampled under and destroyed. This common mistake continues to be made today. This crucial mistake can have far-reaching consequences, especially when the boundaries of the crime scene are extended: when investigators widen their search area and discover that there are multiple crime scenes.

Then there was the questionable reliance by investigators on polygraph tests. Tommy Skakel lied in his first lie detector test, and the results were called inconclusive. These results were then attributed to Tom's emotional stress and to his being extremely tired. He was retested several weeks later and, though still lying about what Martha Moxley and he did that night, he passed. Bruce Atwell, the Skakel family tutor, was under medication when he failed to pass several polygraph tests, yet, as it has turned out, Atwell was telling the truth. Finally, Michael Skakel was never given a polygraph test in the first place. The polygraph is still very overrated by police and investigators. The key insight on this very limited tool is that its evidence is not admissible in most courts of law. Police should understand how and when they should use the lie detector.

Finally, I want to discuss the role in modern criminal justice played by confessions, once the keystone of any successful investigation. Confessions can still play a major role in criminal investigations. Yet, as in the murder of Martha Moxley, Michael Skakel's recurring confessions to this crime over a period of years proved to only be a part of the prosecution's successful case. A couple of years ago, my coauthor, Tom O'Neil, had been sitting in my outer office when a parade of Chinese police officials, starting with an older chief and ending with several very young investigators, came out of my office. When asked, I said that the group was a police command from China, adding that I'd just told them, "It's wrong to beat a confession out of a man. . . . You might be beating a confession out of the wrong man." There is some irony in that statement, though not too many years ago, police in this country, particularly the larger cities, still routinely interrogated defendants to obtain confessions. This "old school" practice has been discarded here, except in very rare instances, and, when exposed, this misconduct invariably leads to a mistrial or even a reversal of a conviction.

A recent book, *Troubling Confessions: Speaking Guilt in Law and Literature,* by Dr. Peter Brooks of Yale University, sheds light on the age-old question of confessions and their value in the criminal justice system.[43] Brooks, to begin his analysis, uses an 1819 Vermont case to establish his point. Two brothers had been feuding with a neighbor, who suddenly disappeared. Though the missing man's body was never found, the pair was convicted of his murder, and the two were then sentenced to hang. The townspeople visited the brothers in their jail cells and urged them to confess so that they would get a better fate in the next life. After some pressure, the brothers admitted to the murder. However, their defense lawyer had been advertising in area papers, asking for any information on the deceased. A few days before the brothers' scheduled execution, word came in that the missing neighbor had only moved to Schenectady, New York, where he was alive and well. Brooks goes on to argue that there are many more ways to coerce a confession out of a suspect than physical torture, sleep deprivation, or other psychological abuse. This coercion blurs the critical fault line between the voluntary telling of what has happened and a person's trying to please his interrogators for one reason or another. Brooks studies the background of the United States Supreme Court's *Miranda* decision, written by Chief Justice Earl Warren in the 1960s. He especially emphasizes the enormous difference between the theoretical treatment of confession, as found in the classroom and in the courtroom, and the way confessions are obtained in the precinct houses of the nation. I do not point any of this out to call into question the repeated confessions of guilt made by Michael Skakel among his peers in the Martha Moxley murder. The quote from lead prosecutor Jonathan Benedict that begins this chapter sums up things very well. In fact, writers and others who followed this case over the years point to Michael Skakel's recurring words as a sign of his deep sense of guilt for the terrible crime he committed in 1975, when he was fifteen. Yet the questions raised about confessions by an increasing number of writers and scholars today only serve, in my scientist's opinion, to underscore the importance that forensic and scientific evidence will play in courtrooms in the years ahead.

THE SUMMARY

It is my experience that most cases that are not solved quickly and that become "cold cases" are the ones in which investigators make critical mistakes from the very outset. Police are human beings and, as such, are as capable of making mistakes as doctors or lawyers or anyone else. The critical mistakes made in the Skakel case were almost all made in the first forty-eight hours following the discovery of Martha Moxley's badly beaten body. Police, however, cannot control or be held accountable for the actions of others, such as the state's chief medical examiner. The timing of the autopsy was one obvious error. Compounding this delay was the medical examiner's holding onto four-color photographs of the corpse, forever denying investigators any chance to determine lividity and other critical factors.

The police department did not properly cordon off the potential crime scenes and otherwise preserve possible evidence on that hillside in Belle Haven where the murder occurred. Beyond that initial error, the department moved into a case it was unprepared to solve in a very defensive manner. Rather than reaching out for assistance from investigators more experienced in this kind of homicide, the department seemed to view the possibility of any outside assistance as a meddlesome and negative comment on their abilities. How would any suburban department inexperienced in homicides be expected to be ready to solve a crime or even properly investigate a murder such as this one? This attitude became a smokescreen behind which cynics could claim that the department had been paid off to go easy on this investigation. Thus the department's resentment of outside assistance only fed the cynical and unfounded conclusion that it was also corrupt. However, the failure to conduct a thorough search of the Skakel house's bathrooms, sinks, and drainpipes for blood evidence was also a mistake that should have been avoided.

Finally, the investigation of the Martha Moxley murder presented a classic example of detectives prematurely narrowing their focus on certain theories of the crime and certain suspects. Michael Skakel escalated this process when he was quick to point out that his brother, Tom, was the last one to see Martha Moxley alive and that he had seen his brother place his hand on her knee, only to have it brushed aside. The police also wasted many valuable man-hours, shortly after the body was found, in tracking down the hundreds of leads they received from the public to their queries about vagrant, would-be killers wandering along the Connecticut Turnpike.

All in all, the Skakel case is full of tragedy. Martha Moxley, as young, vivacious, and delightful a person as she was, is not the only victim of this crime. Her father, David, died before he was sixty. Dorthy and John Moxley are forever scarred by what happened. Within the Skakel family, Tom's life is forever overshadowed by the killing. Tutor Bruce Atwell's career was ruined, and his life was shattered by all of the suspicion of guilt directed at him. And what of the other Skakel children and their father? The tabloids and cynics would have us think that Skakel money mixed with Kennedy power were what was behind the cover-up of the Martha Moxley murder on the night of October 30–31, 1975, and its going unsolved for twenty-seven years. However, applying basic investigative, forensic pathology, and criminalistic skills should have solved this crime many years ago.

CHAPTER THREE

THE JONBENET RAMSEY CASE

A CRY IN THE NIGHT

I had questions all day the day of her death. For hours they [the police] asked us questions trying to get a chronology. I can scarcely recall exactly what happened. They were very compassionate, trying to help us help them. Boulder is a small, peaceful town, unlike Atlanta or New York or LA, where this, God forbid, is a much more frequent occurrence. This does not happen in Boulder. . . . There is a killer on the loose.

—Patsy Ramsey statement during CNN interview
with Brian Cabell on January 1, 1997

The murder of six-year-old JonBenet Ramsey in the early morning of December 26, 1996, remains one of the most perplexing unsolved crimes in recent history. We live in an age of instant and global communication, led by twenty-four-hour-a-day news coverage provided by the media and the Internet. Once the little girl's death became known, this homicide dominated the world media. Set within view of the Rocky Mountains, the picturesque and vibrant college community of Boulder, Colorado, with a population of ninety-five thousand, presented an ironically idyllic backdrop for such a violent crime. The fact that the little victim was a pretty beauty pageant queen only sharpened the interest in this complex and mysterious case, with the net effect that it all seemed to have been scripted. Only the tragic fact was that this heinous crime actually did indeed take place.

The fact that her parents, John and Patsy Ramsey, were quite wealthy, were politically well connected, and lived in a large, opulent house, also served to accelerate the intense firestorm of coverage of this case. Inevitably, given today's culture, journalists flocked to Boulder, many hired by the less-scrupulous tabloid media, and their at-times frenzied reporting poured more gasoline onto this conflagration. Almost overnight, authors and amateur detectives sprang up everywhere, including the Internet, all chiming in with their theories and their renditions of the facts of this case. Since some reports indicate that JonBenet was possibly sexually assaulted before she was killed, fascination increased even among those who do not read the tabloids. Other unhealthy factors also emerged that quickly began to impede the professional pursuit of the truth of JonBenet's death. With the media crawling all over Boulder, investigators and witnesses found themselves perpetually in or near the spotlight. Most directly involved with the investigation were those unfamiliar with the various bargaining tools that a reporter can whisper into a hesitant source's ear, to help elicit a comment or fact. Some individuals, who might have known better had they more experience in a high-profile case, became too open with the media, hiding behind the relative anonymity afforded to them for their "off-the-record" and "not-for-attribution" remarks. Media abuses, particularly from the tabloids, also included ready sums of money in exchange for photographs, information, and hidden microphones. There even loomed the pathetic specter of a tabloid reporter's joining the Ramsey family's Episcopal congregation for weekly services. All of this quickly led to police superiors becoming suspicious of their sister agencies or subordinates leaking stories—a pervasive mind-set that served to undermine departmental morale. More important, the Boulder Police Department circled its wagons in a tight formation, even excluding the Boulder County prosecutor's office from its inner councils. The rift that developed between the prosecutor's office and the Boulder Police Department became as large as any that I have ever experienced. And all of this discord and drama seemed to be in a free fall, without any means or hope of the investigation's beginning to right itself.

Victory has many fathers, but defeat is most often an orphan. In the JonBenet Ramsey case, there was enough blame to go around to cover all of the hundreds of individuals who participated in this investigation. From the very moment when Patsy Ramsey made her 911 call to the Boulder police switchboard, at 5:52 AM on the dark, wintry Thursday of December 26, the investigations into JonBenet's disappearance and death were plagued by severe mistakes. Mrs. Ramsey, in a hysterical state, first reported a suspected kidnapping to the police. Between sobs, she told the dispatcher that JonBenet had been kidnapped from their home at 755 Fifteenth Street on University Hill, less than a mile from the University of Colorado's huge campus. A few moments later, a single patrol officer arrived at the crime scene and briefly searched the large, four-story Tudor-style home. He then read what purported to be a three-page, handwritten ransom note. This long and convoluted message demanded a peculiar amount of ransom money, $118,000. The purported kidnappers claimed they were a small foreign faction, signing off with the initials S.B.T.C. The lone uniformed officer promptly called for backup and, within a few moments, a second patrolman arrived. Two hours then elapsed before the first detective arrived at the scene. During this critical time period, Patsy Ramsey had begun to reach out to her considerably wide circle of close friends, asking them to come over to provide support, and several did. Some wandered through the house. Thus, during this crucial interval, any semblance of a properly secured and protected crime scene disappeared forever into the thin, mountainous air.

These initial, drastic mistakes serve only as a few examples of what was yet to come in the first few hours and days of the JonBenet Ramsey murder investigation. Later in the chapter, I will discuss the continuing nature of the catastrophic missteps that continued to be taken. I will do this with great sadness, in large part because many of the individuals who either allowed or authored these mistakes are conscientious and have dedicated their lives to solving and preventing crimes. Some remain my friends. But I feel compelled to speak out about the terrible way that things went wrong because this case has yet to be solved. Whoever was responsible for the death of JonBenet Ramsey has never been identified or brought before the bar of justice and forced to answer for what he or she has done. The little girl's death is the ultimate tragedy. However, the breakdown in finding the party or parties responsible for her death represents a reprehensible miscarriage of justice—one that may haunt the annals of American criminal justice forever.

THE FACTS OF THE CASE

Like so many others, I first heard about JonBenet Ramsey's death shortly after Christmas in 1996. I do not remember the exact moment with any clarity, but soon, like everyone else, I was watching footage of a very pretty little girl prancing about a stage in a sequin dress, a hat tilted rakishly atop her head, and a cane in her hands. Even prior to her death, many people had already seen Jon-Benet in action at a children's pageant, since she had established herself as a star performer, winning the Little Miss Colorado competition in 1995. Sitting in my study, I could only shake my head in disbelief over the terrible news of what had happened to her. At the time, I was director of the Connecticut State Forensic Science Laboratory in Meriden and was facing my normally heavy caseload. Still, certain facts from the Ramsey case leaped out at me, such as the existence of the three-page, strangely crafted ransom note. It was initially discovered by JonBenet's mother on the steps of a staircase off of the family's kitchen that led to the second floor. Even with all of my state police forensic work and the winter trimester teaching of a graduate class at the University of New Haven, the strange and macabre nature of what I heard sank in and made me think.

I'm taking time to explain my feelings now as a preamble to digging into this very complex case. That's because, to analyze the JonBenet Ramsey case appropriately, we have to also delve into the background of the Ramsey family. While the possibility remains that someone outside the immediate family broke into that home during the night after Christmas, this set of circumstances is a remote possibility. This outside assailant would have to have written the bizarre ransom note, then have sexually assaulted the victim and mortally wounded her with a blow to her head, and finally have garroted her, leaving her body on the cement in a room in the house's cluttered maze of a basement. I will describe the investigative details a little later in this chapter and why I feel so strongly about this case. But suffice it to say for now that there has been no credible evidence found of a forced entry into the Ramsey household, and no footprints were discovered outside any windows or doors providing access to this large house. True, a number of people, friends and family employees, had keys to the Ramsey home, but I am convinced that these individuals have appropriately been eliminated as suspects. That being the case, it is most essential for the investigator to analyze closely the backgrounds of JonBenet's parents, how that tragic day unfolded, and what their relationship was like with their surviving son, Burke, who was nine the night that his younger sister was murdered.

John and Patricia Ramsey moved from Atlanta to Boulder in 1991, after Mr. Ramsey had merged Access Graphics—the computer distribution and service company he had started in 1980—with two other corporations, one from New Jersey and the other already in Boulder. As president of this new and expanded enterprise, John Ramsey's even-tempered yet energetic style set a tone for the company's excellent reputation. In late 1996, Access Graphics passed the $1 billion mark in gross sales, a fact that Patsy Ramsey proudly played up in the family's annual Christmas newsletter. Access Graphics's key strength was its ability to provide its worldwide business clients with outstanding computer hardware and software pack-

ages. All this was backed up, most essentially, by a team of very conscientious support experts, who educated and otherwise assisted
employees at client companies in establishing computer networks,
then in maximizing the output and quality of work from their computer systems. As the corporation's customer base thrived, word
quickly spread through the computer marketplace that this distributor in Boulder was the place to go, especially to solve difficult problems. Access Graphics thus flourished accordingly, attracting many
bright newcomers to its employee ranks. Very little further testament
has to be accorded John Ramsey's intelligence and work ethic. Only
a person whose mind was disciplined and focused could accomplish
all of this. Ramsey also knew how to reach out to those he most inti-
mately trusted to help Access Graphics. Donald Paugh, Patsy
Ramsey's father, regularly commuted to Boulder from his home in
Atlanta so he could take care of personnel matters and other administrative details for his son-in-law. A retired engineer, Don Paugh
had spent the bulk of his career at Union Carbide in West Virginia,
where he'd become a successful manager. When Paugh would travel
west, Patsy's mother, Nedra, held down the family household back
in the Atlanta area, busying herself with the couple's other two
grown daughters, Pamela and Paulette, and their families.[1]

Patricia Ann Paugh was born on December 29, 1956, in Parkersburg, West Virginia. Called "Patsy" from birth by her family, she was
the oldest of the family's three daughters. Her father was an engineering graduate from the University of West Virginia, who in 1955
married his Ritchie County high school sweetheart, Nedra Rymer,
while he was still in the army. After his honorable discharge, the
couple settled into Parkersburg in neighboring Wood County, where
Don had taken his first job at Bendix Westinghouse. Nedra, who
came from a large family, had been a cheerleader in high school, as
were two of her older sisters, and this probably whetted her lifelong
interest in public performance. By the time Patsy Paugh was four,
she was prancing before audiences in little costumes very similar to
those JonBenet wore thirty-five years later. Bright, very effervescent,
with her pretty face ringed by her black hair, Patsy became a star in
her grade school and high school years, winning debating titles as

well as beauty contests. Patsy's activities and awards added up to a full page in her high school yearbook. In 1975 she entered West Virginia University, where she continued to dazzle both her professors and classmates. Majoring in journalism, with a minor in marketing, Patsy also set out to compete for the title of Miss America. In 1976, after her freshman year, she traveled to Atlantic City, where the national competition is annually staged, to take notes on how to succeed. The following year, Patsy won the title of Miss West Virginia, which included her coveted ticket to Atlantic City for the nationally televised Miss America pageant. Though she did not win the ultimate prize of becoming Miss America, Patsy did herself proud at the competition. She finished in the top five contestants, giving her even more flattering national exposure. After returning to school that fall to continue working toward her degree, Patsy proved so good at the public appearances as the reigning Miss West Virginia that she quickly found herself offered public relations jobs that became her summer work. Yet her family and friends attest to the fact that all of this did not go to Patsy's head as she completed her final two years in Morgantown, earning her degree, magna cum laude, in June of 1979.

Following her graduation in 1979, Patsy and a girlfriend moved to the Atlanta area. They quickly became part of the circle of young and single adults, a crowd that centered around one of the newer and posher apartment complexes that had sprouted up to accommodate the thousands of successful young professionals who'd flocked there. Sitting around their pool, Patsy met John Ramsey, an attractive and recently divorced businessman who had just started his own computer company. He was also the father of three children and was thirteen years older than his future wife. John Bennett Ramsey had been born in Omaha, Nebraska, the second son of James Ramsey, a decorated World War II pilot, and his wife, Mary Jane. When he was thirteen, the family had moved to Okemas, Michigan, a farming town near Lansing. In 1961 John entered nearby Michigan State University, where he met Lucinda Lou Pasch, a pretty coed whom he would marry in 1966, the year he graduated with an electrical engineering degree. A member of the university's naval ROTC program, Ramsey was commissioned an ensign and served two years in the engineering corps, a tour of duty that took him to Subic Bay in the Philippine Islands. After his navy service, Ramsey went back to Michigan State for a master's degree and finally in the early seventies resettled his family in Atlanta.

Atlanta had become the principal city of the New South, and there John Ramsey, now sporting a trim, attractive beard, found himself drawn to the skyrocketing computer field. By the end of the seventies, he'd already started one small company, called Microsouth, a software distributor. Very unassuming, John drove a beat-up pickup truck that was fifteen years old. For recreation, nonetheless, he got his pilot's license and flew quite often. However, things were not going smoothly in John Ramsey's married life, perhaps because of the backbreaking hours that he worked. Finally, in 1978, Lucinda and John Ramsey filed for divorce. The couple's three children, Elizabeth, Melinda, and John Andrew, lived with their mother, who remained in the Atlanta area, and John, a very conscientious father, stayed in close touch with all three. In Linda Edison McLean's book *JonBenet's Mother: The Tragedy and the Truth!* a friend of Patsy Ramsey's, who had known her for twenty years, described a dinner party that John and Patsy attended together early in their dating relationship. At exactly eight that evening, John excused himself from the table and disappeared for twenty minutes. The three left at the table wondered if their boisterous behavior had bothered their quiet companion. Not so. John had used the interval to make his daily call to his children. Later on, Patsy and her friend came to expect this daily ritual from John. Ramsey's very quiet manner presented a sharp contrast to Patsy's outgoing humor, yet the two got along very well, and they married in 1980.[2] It should be noted that before John met Patsy, he and Jim Marino, an employee of John's first company, would go out to socialize in places where they could meet attractive and unattached young women. In a 1997 interview in *People* magazine, Marino said that any and all of that activity by John stopped once he had met Patsy Paugh.[3]

After their wedding, Patsy and John settled into a home of their own and became very active in their church, where they met and mingled with other young adults. When they were first married, John used his home's basement as his office, and Patsy answered the phone. The couple's first child, a son named Burke, was born in 1987, and JonBenet followed in 1990. Patsy became quite close to her husband's three children from his first marriage, and the couple got along well with the former Mrs. Ramsey and her second husband. Often, all five children and their parents got together for the holidays. Still, John was very busy building Access Graphics and was on the road a good deal of the time, preparing his company for the coming mergers and its growth. Before having children, Patsy kept busy with her widening circle of friends from the church groups with whom she sometimes traveled out of state for weekends. Mrs. Ramsey also attended to the social duties of a corporate wife, an increasing responsibility for her as Access Graphics continued to thrive and expand. Then, in 1991, the company's two mergers required the family to relocate to Boulder, a location that must have reminded John of his happy years spent in East Lansing. There the very successful couple bought their fifteen-room home on University Hill.

As the family adjusted to their new Colorado surroundings, providing a wealthier lifestyle than any of them had ever known, the Ramseys were able to enjoy the success that John's prosperity afforded them. They purchased a rustic vacation home on a lake in Charlevoix, Michigan, in the upper portion of that state that is famous for its beautiful summers. They found it an ideal spot for getting all five children together, along with Patsy's parents and her two sisters, who had also married and had their own children. John acquired a sailboat while he was up there. Yet with all of this success and joy, a tragedy lay just on the horizon for John and Patsy. In early 1992 John's oldest child, Elizabeth, and her boyfriend were both killed in an auto accident in the Chicago area. This tragedy devastated the Ramsey family and, quite naturally, hit John the hardest. Rather than find an immediate escape in his work, John's attention to his corporate duties seemed to slip a bit. However, the challenges that Access Graphics presented proved a blessing to John, and he was soon able to regain his corporate focus and find an escape in his work. This included his selling control of his Access Graphics to the corporate giant, Lockheed Martin, a move that made John and Patsy Ramsey multimillionaires. With all of John Ramsey's accomplishments, just as he seemed to be coming to terms with the loss of Elizabeth, his father died. This new tragedy seemed to reopen the wounds that Ramsey had suffered over her death. Ramsey again seemed to disappear into himself and then his work.

Since their move to Boulder, Patsy Ramsey dedicated her very considerable energies to adding on rooms and otherwise improving the couple's house. Friends joked that, with all the renovations, John wasn't able to find their master bedroom, which Patsy had moved to the house's third floor. JonBenet's and Burke's rooms were on the spacious second floor, with hers close to the narrow and winding stairs that led to the parents' bedroom on the third floor. Two other second-floor bedrooms were set aside for John's two surviving children from his first marriage: Melinda, for when she visited from Atlanta, where she worked as a nurse, and John Andrew, who had matriculated to the University of Colorado as a sophomore and regularly came to visit there.

As 1993 started, the family suffered another staggering blow when Patsy was diagnosed with an advanced case of ovarian cancer, a disease that had spread to her lymph nodes and had become lymphoma. At least one doctor told John Ramsey that there was nothing that could be done. Because of the critical status of her cancer, Patsy enrolled in an experimental study at the National Cancer Institute in the Washington, DC, area, a decision driven by John's intensive research. Every three weeks Patsy traveled to Bethesda, Maryland, to receive a powerful combination of drugs. Slowly, her chemotherapy began to make progress in beating back the two forms of cancer in her system. At the same time, the chemo brought for Patsy its common side effects, a loss of strength, the loss of her hair, and severe bouts with nausea. Patsy told friends that her parents, husband, children, and God were the sources of the strength she showed as she slowly began to conquer the disease. John became quieter than usual during this critical period, and some have said that the couple was not as openly affectionate toward one another as they had been. While Patsy was extremely ill for almost half a year, her mother, Nedra, looked after the two children. The family tried to maintain a normal life as best they could. They spent the summer in Charlevoix, as usual. Finally, in 1995, Patsy was given a clean bill of health. She had beaten two lethal forms of cancer.[4]

At five, JonBenet was old enough to intuit that her mother had been in grave danger. Though outwardly as positive as her parents and older brother, her distress caused the child to slip severely in her toilet training. She became a constant bed wetter, to her mother's consternation. The pretty little girl with long blond locks also would soil herself when she was out in public, and she made it a habit of asking any available adult to clean her up. This practice worried John and Patsy, and they were not always able to stop JonBenet from turning to outsiders for this kind of intimate help. Moreover, this child possessed a surprisingly mature ability to express herself and otherwise deal with adults. Lawrence Schiller, in his very comprehensive book *Perfect Murder, Perfect Town—JonBenet and the City of Boulder*, relates how Brian Scott, the Ramsey family's gardener, carried on complicated conversations with JonBenet. In a written account of one conversation, Scott recalled JonBenet asking him, "Do roses know their thorns can hurt?"[5]

With Patsy's health restored, she threw herself into her daughter's life with renewed vigor and with the family's considerable economic resources. Access Graphics's dramatic growth meant that John was a millionaire, several times over. If the Ramseys decided to get behind a project, they went for it all the way. John and Patsy both actively supported the formation of an elementary charter school in their section of Boulder that other area parents had already started to plan. This effort culminated in the fall of 1995 with the opening of High Peaks Elementary School. Burke Ramsey enrolled in the third grade and JonBenet entered its prekindergarten program. Besides financial help, Patsy Ramsey became a tireless volunteer at the school, which depended heavily on its parents for their enthusiasm and assistance. John and Patsy Ramsey were also very active at the St. John's Episcopal Church in Boulder, where they were known for pledging financial assistance. The Ramseys' successful lifestyle also included more summer trips to their place in Michigan and a trip to the 1996 Olympic Games in Atlanta.

Besides starting JonBenet at school, Patsy Ramsey introduced her daughter to the world of child beauty pageants. The five-year-old seemed "a natural," spontaneously moving about the stage during her first performances and through long periods of rehearsal. Jonny B, as the family and a few close friends liked to call her, was heartily encouraged in her fledgling theatrical career by Patsy and by her grandmother, Nedra. Called "a stage mother" by family friends, Nedra even liked to refer to JonBenet as her "future Miss America."[6] Things in the pageant world began to get very serious in 1995, when Patsy took JonBenet to a dance studio in Westminster, twenty miles southeast of Boulder. Renee Walter* had been a Broadway dancer, appearing in *Hello, Dolly!* and other huge shows, and Patsy retained her to work with JonBenet three times a week. Renee had been referred to the Ramseys by their seamstress, Ellen Howard* of Longmont, twenty miles northeast of Boulder, whose daughter, Penny,* a high school senior, had started training JonBenet on how to impress the judges as she strutted down a runway. As a little girl, Penny had won several competitions, bringing her a beauty queen's shiny crown, a trophy she showed Patsy and JonBenet. In addition, Patsy was beginning to reach out to photographers in the Boulder area to create a portfolio for her daughter. Ellen Howard particularly recommended one located in Boulder, Herb Andrews,* whose specialty was making very young children look twenty. Patsy Ramsey was putting her enormous energy and finances behind her only daughter's promising pageant career. JonBenet herself never showed any reluctance to put in the demanding hours for rehearsals or for performing in front of strangers, according to this new circle of coaches and other supporters. All of this effort ultimately led to JonBenet's winning the Little Miss Colorado title in July of 1995 in the Gingerbread Productions of America competition. Later that summer, Patsy passed on JonBenet entering an early-September national competition in Atlanta, since the dates conflicted with a family outing, and for Mrs. Ramsey, family came first. John Ramsey also balked at the possibility of JonBenet entering a national competition that was moving to Las Vegas, since he didn't want his daughter exposed to the culture there. Patsy Ramsey later on tried to dismiss the otherwise challenging rehearsal, preps, and pageant schedule as taking up just a few Sundays, a denial that likely had a hollow ring to it.

In addition to the bed-wetting, JonBenet exhibited some other signs of stress. In the last three years she lived in Boulder, the little girl had to go to her pediatrician's office a total of twenty-times, or about once every six weeks. Perhaps because she spent many nights sleeping between urine-soaked and cold sheets, JonBenet often had problems with her throat, coughing incessantly and spitting up mucus. She also complained about irritations in her vaginal area, brought on, the pediatrician decided, by an overabundance of bubble baths. JonBenet's doctor said that even that high number of visits to his office was not that unusual for a girl her age, and, when later asked, he also said there was no evidence of any kind of sexual abuse. It appeared that JonBenet's relationship with her family was good, and she seemed particularly close to her father, hanging on to his every word and expressing strong resentment that his job required him to be away a good deal of the time. If anything, JonBenet's participation in regional pageants seemed to give her a good deal of pleasure, as well as providing her with all kinds of goals. By now a kindergartner, she continued to improve her singing, dancing, and stage presence. Her grandmother, Nedra, suggested that JonBenet dress for one show looking like a Las Vegas showgirl. With its plumes and obviously provocative approach, this costume created a terrible reaction and, seeing this instant negative response, Patsy quickly put that routine to rest. Still, most of what JonBenet was doing on stage *seemed* very natural for her, culminating in her winning the Little Miss Colorado competition. This exquisitely pretty, blond little girl had received much national television news coverage. Yet the images of JonBenet, dancing in scanty outfits, her face made up to look years older than her actual age, caused many viewers to shake their heads with a kind of sadness.

As the Christmas season of 1996 approached, Patsy Ramsey took the step of getting her large and lavishly decorated home established on an annual fund-raising tour of the especially beautiful homes of Boulder that was sponsored by a local civic organization. Always one to go to the limit, Patsy had purchased, decorated, and placed in each bedroom an individual Christmas tree. Yards of festive green and red bunting adorned the banisters and staircases. The exterior of the house sparkled under the glow of hundreds of lights and a huge tree, illuminated with scores of outdoor bulbs. Red-and-white wooden candy canes bordered either side of the front walkway. The home's large living room fireplace was framed with gay Christmas decorations in a room dominated by a huge and beautiful holiday tree set off near the entrance foyer. Mistletoe and other cheery Christmas ornaments seemed to dangle everywhere. In the pre-Christmas days of December, thousands of local residents and their out-of-town guests wandered through the Ramseys' beautifully fes-tooned home to gaze at and admire its beauty. None of these indi-viduals, however, was invited downstairs, into the basement. This space was a maze of clutter. According to Patsy's maid and others who worked at the Ramsey house, whenever Patsy didn't know what to do with an object, she consigned it to the concrete-floored base-ment. Boxes of books and video games, as well as old clothing and bicycles, were everywhere. This basement-as-the-catch-all area became so pronounced that it was something of an unspoken household joke. The net effect was a basement space that was very difficult to navigate, especially since, by design, it contained a number of very small rooms that had no apparent purpose, such as a small, empty room located behind the house's furnace, referred to as the wine cellar. Further complicating navigation in the Ramsey basement was the fact that there was no single lighting switch any-where that could illuminate its dark interior. Anyone moving about down there had to move from one localized light switch to the next.

John and Patsy Ramsey threw a Christmas party for their friends the evening of Monday, December 23. None of these guests was from Access Graphics, since John Ramsey liked to keep his work and personal life very separate. JonBenet helped the arriving neighbors and other guests by taking their coats. Each family at the party was given a gingerbread house to decorate with gumdrops. A Santa Claus moved about, providing good humor. In actuality, this individual was Austin O'Rourke,* a retired professor of journalism from the university who had known the Ramseys since shortly after they had moved to Boulder in 1991. O'Rourke was a trusted friend, particularly of Patsy's, and, because he was over quite often to provide help as a handyman, he had a key to the house. Sanford Lucas* was a guest, along with his wife, Renee,* and her parents. Lucas, a very successful businessman in the oil field, was a particularly close friend of John Ramsey's. Out of this happy party, though, a grim omen emerged. Something was said to JonBenet that evening that later would be closely scrutinized. This came to light the following day, Christmas Eve, when JonBenet was at the home of a young playmate. There she told her girlfriend and the child's mother that she'd already seen and talked directly to Santa Claus, who'd been at her family's party the previous evening. Santa had promised JonBenet that he'd be over to her house late Christmas night when he was going to give her a very special present. The listening mother misunderstood what she'd just heard and tried to correct JonBenet. The parent replied that JonBenet must have meant late that very night, since Christmas Eve was when Santa visited everyone's home. No, JonBenet insisted, Santa Claus had promised her the visit and the present later on, on Christmas night itself.

When Christmas morning dawned, the Ramseys awoke, went downstairs, and exchanged their gifts. Melinda and John Andrew were then driven to the Denver airport, to return home to Atlanta to celebrate the rest of the holiday with their mother and her family. At 4:30 in the afternoon, the Ramseys went over to the Lucases' house, where they had Christmas dinner, along with another couple, and Renee's sister and her boyfriend. After dinner, the party moved to the living room, where all eight adults got down on the carpeted floor and played games. Neighbors later joined the festivities for some Christmas caroling. Around 9:30 that evening, the Ramseys left to visit two other families and to drop off gifts, and around 11:00, they returned home. There are very few other established facts about exactly what happened over the course of the next seven hours. Late that night, just as a neighbor across the street was dozing off, she heard a horrific scream from the Ramsey house, one loud enough to penetrate her own partially open bedroom window. Hearing nothing more, this neighbor fell into a deep sleep.

THE INVESTIGATION OF THE CASE

The investigation into the death of JonBenet Ramsey carries with it many complexities. Some of these are due to tragic mistakes made by the investigators themselves. Given the controversy and the gaudily public nature of this case, it is most important that I present the facts, as I know them, with as much clarity as possible. To do this, I have decided to present a detailed timeline for what happened on Thursday, December 26, 1996, from the very first morning and midday of the Ramsey investigation. Rather than just present a simple outline, I will provide the times and factual information along with my own insights:

5:45 AM (approx.)—According to Patsy Ramsey, after applying her makeup, she left her third-floor master bedroom and descended a spiral staircase to the second floor. There, she washed JonBenet's soiled jumpsuit that she'd found in a laundry space just opposite her bedroom. She did not open the doors to either her daughter's bedroom or to her son's, which was next door. Finishing this chore, Patsy descended the spiral stairs, and, just a step above the kitchen floor, she found a handwritten note on three pages that came from a white, lined stationery pad. Without stepping on these pages, she quickly determined that this was a ransom note about JonBenet, and she dashed back upstairs to discover her daughter missing from her bed, and then she screamed for her husband.

5:52 AM—Patsy Ramsey dialed 911 and told the Boulder Police Department's dispatcher that her daughter, JonBenet, was missing and had been kidnapped. She mentioned a ransom note. Her husband, John, was with her when she, in a voice bordering on the hysterical, made this report. In her distraught condition, Mrs. Ramsey failed to place the telephone directly into its cradle, and the line was open for a few more seconds.

5:56 AM (approx.)—Uniformed officer Rick French arrived at the Ramsey home and quickly made a search of the house, but he found no sign of the missing girl and no sign of a forced entry into the home. The Ramseys then showed him what purported to be a ransom note, one Mrs. Ramsey said she found lying in three handwritten pages on the bottom steps that led down from the second floor to her kitchen. Officer French quickly read the 368-word document, addressed to only John Ramsey. It said that it was left by an international faction calling itself the S.B.T.C., signed off with it under the slogan "Victory!" These kidnappers threatened JonBenet with a quick death by beheading unless they received $118,000 in unmarked bills ($100,000 in hundred dollar bills and the final $18,000 in twenties), or if the parents or anyone else notified the police, the FBI, or others. The note's authors also promised they were going to get back to Jon-Benet's parents at the Ramsey home by telephone with further instructions between eight and ten later that morning. Patsy Ramsey told Officer French that John Ramsey had gotten up before her that morning, around 5:30, and had taken his shower. French then called for backup.

6:10 AM (approx.)—A second uniformed officer, Karl Veitch, arrived at the house. Mr. and Mrs. Ramsey, in their distress, had been frantically calling friends to report this disaster, and, by this time, some of them had begun to arrive to offer the Ramseys comfort and assistance. Three additional uniformed officers were called to go to the house, and four detectives were then paged. Sgt. Bob Whitson was the on-duty watch commander. Many key people were on vacation, including Det. Sgt. Larry Mason and his boss, Cdr. John Eller, head of the detective division. There was only a skeleton crew on duty at the Boulder Police Department on the morning of this phone call, the day after Christmas.

6:40 AM (approx.)—Sergeant Whitson recalled that during that year the Boulder department had sent a detective to the FBI's Child Abduction Serial Killer Unit for training and that she had returned with a manual for dealing with cases like this. However, she, too, was on vacation, and Whitson did not know how to contact her or where she had stored the FBI's suggested protocol for such cases. He then remembered that a lieutenant in the Boulder County Sheriff's Department had also attended this training. He contacted him. Meanwhile, Boulder police sergeant Paul Reichenbach, and Officers Barry Weiss and Sue Barcklow arrived at the Ramsey home.

7:10 AM (approx.)—Sgt. Whitson received a copy of the FBI manual. He quickly consulted it, though the Boulder Police Department had not yet adopted its recommendations as official policy. Back at the Ramsey house, John Ramsey awakened his son, Burke, and quickly made arrangements for him to be taken by Sanford Lucas and another friend, Frank Torrell,* to spend the day at Lucas's home. Ramsey also phoned his personal broker and friend, Hugh Averill,* at his home in Atlanta, where business hours had already begun. He told Averill what had happened and that he would need a substantial amount of cash. Averill immediately started to make arrangements to transfer the money to a Boulder bank from a cash management account of Ramsey's that had more than a million dollars in it.

8:10 AM—Boulder police detectives Linda Arndt and Fred Patterson arrived at the Ramsey household and found a number of persons milling about the crime scene. These people

included Renee and Sanford Lucas, Frank and Denise Torrell,* (another couple with whom Mr. and Mrs. Ramsey were
very friendly), the Reverend Rol Hoverstock (the minister of
the Ramseys' church), and even two victims' advocates, who
were automatically summoned to a major crime scene by the
Boulder police. Thus, by the time detectives arrived at the
crime scene, a number of people had been freely coming and
going about for more than an hour or two. Some time after
the detectives' arrival, Sanford Lucas, on his own initiative,
went down into the Ramseys' basement and looked around,
opening the doors to its several smaller rooms and peering
inside these extra chambers. Detective Patterson questioned
the Ramseys on what had happened when they awoke that
morning. He was told that Burke Ramsey, JonBenet's older
brother, had slept through the discovery of the ransom note
and through Patsy's highly emotional 911 call.

8:20 AM (approx.)—Det. Linda Arndt, who had a reputation
within the department for treating individuals at crime
scenes in a compassionate manner, quickly assessed matters
at the Ramsey house and called for more backup. She saw
that Patsy Ramsey was very close to being totally out of control. As the minutes passed, Arndt also noticed that John and
Patsy Ramsey did not sit together or spend a lot of time con-
soling one another. Mrs. Ramsey kept saying "Oh, please let
her be safe," over and over again, and John Ramsey blamed
himself for not setting a burglar alarm on Christmas night.
Arndt read the ransom note and then sent Patrolman Veitch
to police headquarters to book the ransom note as evidence.
Arndt also directed Veitch to show the note to the FBI investigators as soon as they arrived. Arndt and Patterson
instructed Mr. Ramsey to answer all telephone calls and to
stall the kidnappers by claiming that he could not get the
money they demanded until 5:00 PM that afternoon. Then
the police ordered a tap on the Ramsey phone, a device that
collected data from the phone company of any caller or

caller ID and of the identity of any other parties associated with a particular number. Police began searching JonBenet's bedroom and started dusting for fingerprints there. Officer Barry Weiss noticed a large, police-style flashlight on the Ramseys' kitchen counter.

It seems timely here to closely analyze the ransom note (the text of which is in the appendix). This was written on white, lined paper, a note pad eight and a half by eleven inches in size. This rambling communiqué seems very strange, even bizarre, when one remembers its purported heinous purpose. First is its length. Ransom notes are classically very short. At 368 words, this one seems the *Moby Dick* of its genre. In fact, about the only thing right about the note is that it is not written in a business letter format. There is, for instance, no date. In point of fact, the note refers to "tomorrow" as the time for John Ramsey to act to save his daughter, meaning that the author wrote the note before midnight on Wednesday, or wanted readers to think so.

Another most obvious irregularity in the note is the very strange sum of money being demanded by the kidnappers: $118,000. This is a very odd sum for kidnappers to be demanding. Further compounding this strange amount was the fact that this peculiar sum is very close, almost to the dollar, to John Ramsey's year-end bonus from Access Graphics. The odds are very long that the authors, who claim they are part of "a small foreign faction," simply came up with that amount out of the blue. Also, if you consider that Ramsey is later called "a fat cat" by the kidnappers, this seems a modest amount of money to be demanding. Someone of John Ramsey's stature in the business community could have been targeted for several times that amount. So the kidnap note was in all probability authored by individuals quite familiar with the inner workings of the high command at Access Graphics. A very stupid mistake. Unless, of course, the person or persons writing the note wanted to throw open to the police a wide and very specific circle of suspects, individuals at John Ramsey's corporation who knew the firm's otherwise confidential personnel pay structure. In that case, the amount set is a very bright move. There are several other indications in the note that make the entire work appear contrived. The text, even with all its twists and turns, is well laid out, the writing of a well-educated individual. Yet, in only the second line, the authors misspell a simple word: "bussiness." This could then be another ruse. At another point, the note mentions "an earlier delivery of the money," yet goes on to talk about "a earlier" delivery of the little girl to her parents, the type of spelling error that is so obvious that it seems contrived. This second mistake stands out even more when it's noted that the second use of the term "delivery" is crossed out and replaced by the words "a pick-up" of JonBenet. These mistakes are very inconsistent with the rest of the note, and both smack of an attempt to make the authors appear uneducated, individuals perhaps struggling with their English.

Besides referring to John Ramsey's wealth, the authors of the note also go out of their way to confront JonBenet's father on a personal level. The two men actually holding Ramsey's daughter as a hostage "do not particularly like you," the note warns. The kidnappers repeat their warnings, four times, that, if anything goes wrong, "she dies," even by beheading. They then threaten Ramsey that he may never recover his dead daughter's remains, so that the family would never have a "proper burial." At the end of the note, the kidnappers warn Ramsey, "don't try to grow a brain," and implore him to "use that good southern common sense of yours." The writers seem to want readers to understand that they know Ramsey on an intimate level. All of this language also smacks of theatrics. This ransom note is supposed to be about getting $118,000 from John Ramsey in exchange for his daughter. So why would the kidnappers, who know how to write in clear English, bother with personal grudges? Unless, of course, the writer or writers of the note are only trying to look like a vengeful foreign faction.

8:30 AM (approx.)—John Ramsey phoned his office and talked to Eugene Stallworth,* his vice president for human resources. "My daughter's been kidnapped," he told Stallworth. Police later became suspicious that Ramsey was willing to break the kidnappers' orders about telling any outside parties that JonBenet had been kidnapped. Ramsey also willingly made the same statement in a call to the pilot of his private plane and in calls to several others. Following the call to Access Graphics, Boulder police detectives were in Stallworth's office within the hour, asking him about anyone at the corporation who might have had a vendetta against his boss. Stallworth mentioned Todd Ogilvy,* who had been an old friend of John Ramsey's but had been laid off, and Wendy Goodall,* who owed the company a substantial amount of money. The detectives left after warning Stallworth not to mention anything about their interview to anyone, particularly other employees. Back at the Ramsey house, Patsy told Linda Arndt about Arlene Beckworth,* her household maid. Beckworth, who had a key to the house, had been experiencing financial problems. Patsy had recently agreed to lend her $2,000 to help her pay her rent and had planned to write her a check later that day. Beckworth was due to work the next morning. Patsy Ramsey gave police Beckworth's signature on her canceled checks to provide them with her maid's handwriting sample.

9:45 AM (approx.)—Det. Sgt. Larry Mason received an electronic page meant for Sgt. Robert Whitson indicating that FBI agents were at police headquarters and looking for Whitson. This page should have been for Mason, since he was next up the chain of command for a call that morning. Detective Sergeant Mason quickly phoned in and, hearing about the kidnapping, headed for his office at police headquarters, about a half hour away. John Ramsey went down to the basement of his home, where Officer French had conducted an earlier search and where Ramsey then found a window open in Burke's train room. He closed the window. The kidnappers did not call by ten, as their note had promised. At the Ramsey home, police found a roll of undeveloped film and took it to a nearby photo store, where it would be processed by noon.

10:15 AM (approx.)—Detective Sergeant Mason arrived at police headquarters and met with FBI special agent Ron Walker and a four-member team that had just arrived from the bureau's office in Denver, twenty-five miles away. The FBI was busy setting up telephone line taps and traps. Agent Walker, an expert in profiling, was skeptical about the ransom note he'd read, but, for the time being, was going straight ahead, handling the case as an abduction. Lawrence Schiller, in his book *Perfect Murder, Perfect Town,* writes that Walker was particularly concerned with the note's length and the oddball amount being demanded.[7] At the crime scene, John Ramsey provided police with his own and his wife's handwriting samples. He gave police shopping lists and writing on a lined, white stationery pad, similar to the one used for the ransom note. If this request made either parent nervous, since it carried with it an implication of suspicion, neither one showed any concern. Patsy Ramsey continued alternately to weep and talk to no one in particular, repeating "Why did they do this?" as a mantra.

10:30 AM—Det. Fred Patterson ordered JonBenet's bedroom sealed. Det. Linda Arndt and he ordered the house cleared of all nonessential police personnel. Six officers left, and Patterson went to police headquarters to brief Cdr. John Eller on developments. The detectives ordered that the Ramseys and their friends, the Lucases and the Torrells, the Reverend Hoverstock, and the two victim advocates all be placed in a first-floor study at the rear of the house, behind the kitchen. Detective Arndt was now the only police officer present. In just a few minutes, Arndt recognized a problem: she was attempting to ride herd on nine adults, two of whom owned the fifteen-bedroom house. Patsy Ramsey was in great emotional distress, vomiting, and close to fainting. Arndt paged Det. Sgt. Larry Mason and urged backup. Mason found that the few detectives on duty were assigned to other duties on the Ramsey case. For the next two and a half hours, Arndt was the only police presence at the Ramsey house. Mason also discovered that Commander Eller had ordered that Patsy and John Ramsey be treated as victims and not as suspects. Thus, the couple had not been separated and was not being questioned by teams of detectives. Eller later explained to Mason that this was "an influential family."[8]

11:45 AM (approx.)—At police headquarters, Larry Mason suggested to Commander Eller that tracking dogs be used at the Ramsey house to attempt to locate the missing girl. Eller had originally been unclear as to why Mason was at headquarters, forgetting for the moment that the detective was on call. The two men debated the merits of the dogs in the Boulder department that were ground hunters and the possible use of a bloodhound named Yogi from the nearby Aurora Police Department that was an air tracker. In 1993, Yogi was able to find the body of a kidnapped five-year-old girl, who had been transported much of the way in a vehicle. He wasn't as easily distracted as the local dogs, German shepherds. Most likely, Mason pressed, JonBenet had been driven away from her house.

12:55 PM (approx.)—Linda Arndt, still alone at the crime scene, suggested to Sanford Lucas and Frank Torrell that the two friends take John Ramsey on a tour of the house. Arndt had noticed that Ramsey had been getting increasingly despondent, while he waited for the kidnappers' phone call. She asked Ramsey to look for anything of JonBenet's that might be missing. Lucas and Ramsey went down into the basement, while Torrell stayed upstairs. They went into Burke's train room, and Ramsey told Lucas about how he'd had to break the window there to crawl into his house a few months earlier, when he'd locked himself out. There was a suitcase below the broken window, with shards of glass on the floor and some scuffmarks above the suitcase. Then Ramsey walked into the boiler room. Lucas followed his

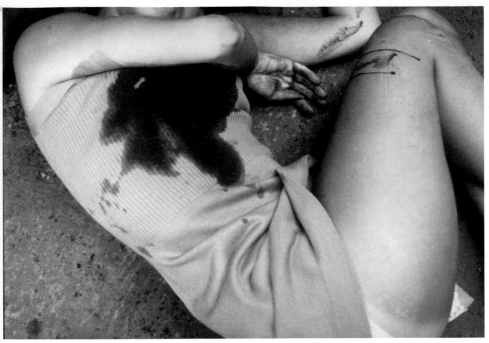

Penney Serra's body was found in the tenth-floor stairwell of the parking garage.

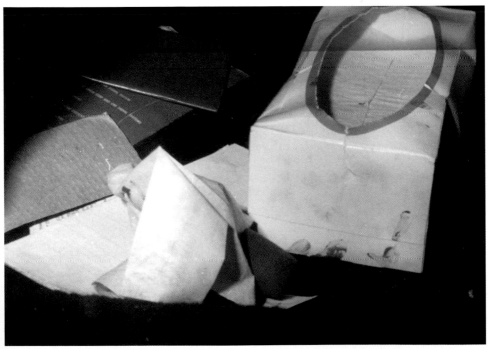

A tissue box was found in the back seat of Penney Serra's car.

All photos are the property of Dr. Lee.

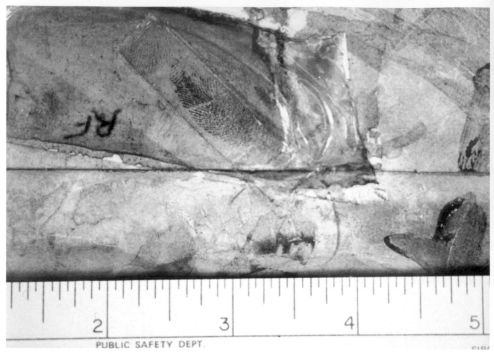

PUBLIC SAFETY DEPT.

Bloody fingerprints were found on the tissue box in the Serra car after chemical enhancement.

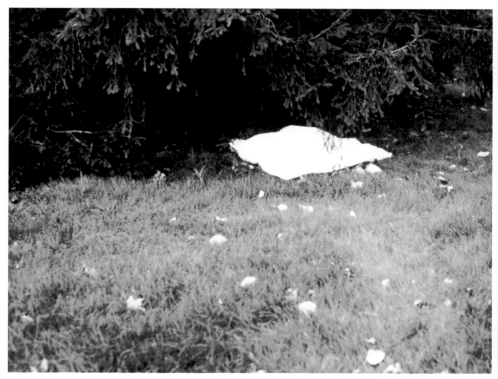

A sheet partially covers Martha Moxley's body found in the backyard.

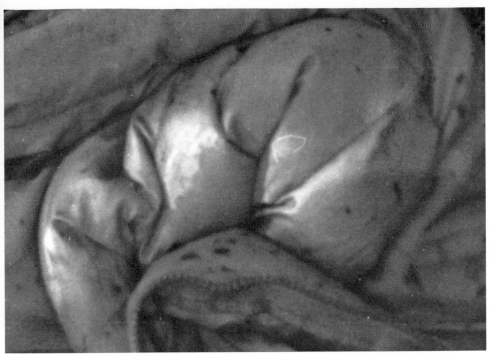

Bloodstains found on Martha Moxley's jacket.

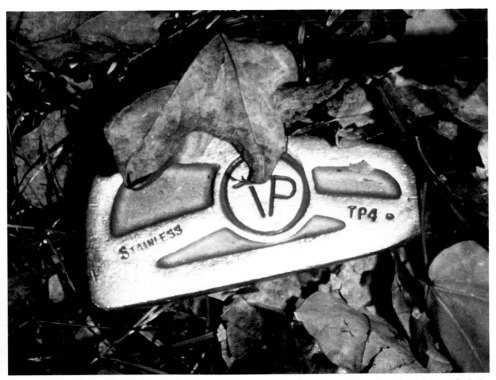

The murder weapon in the Moxley-Skakel case—the head portion of a six iron golf club.

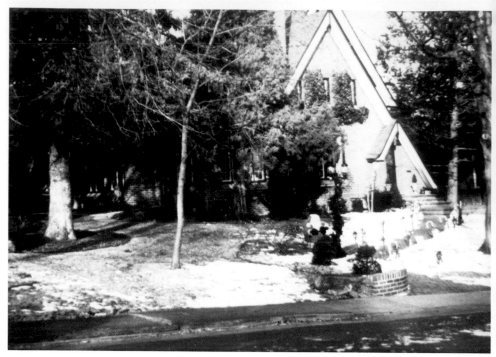

Outside view of the Ramsey house.

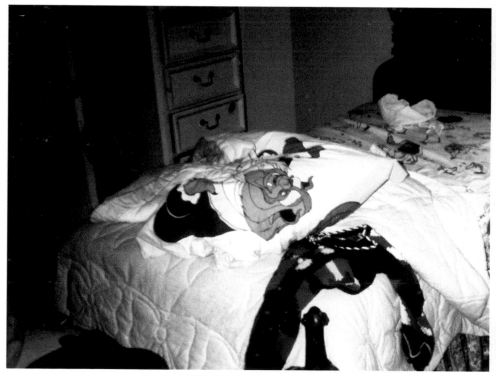

A view of JonBenet Ramsey's bedroom

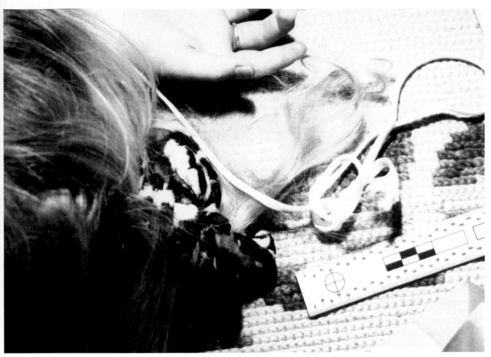

The ligature tied around JonBenet Ramsey's neck and right wrist.

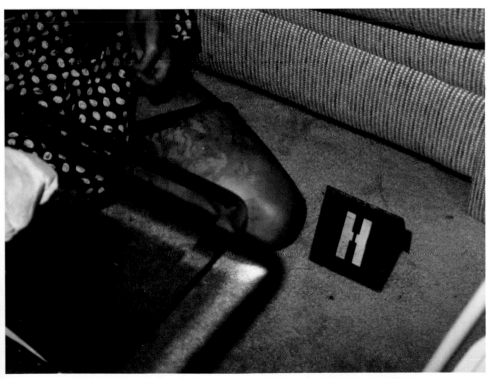

Jennifer Ji's body was found in the living room next to the sofa.

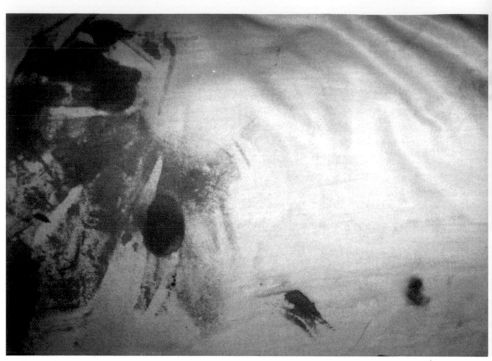

A large bloody handprint was found on the pillow on the sofa in Jennifer Ji's apartment.

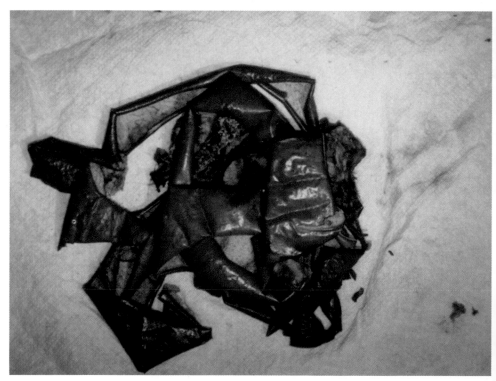

An apple peel was found in the kitchen garbage can at the crime scene in the Lisa Peng case.

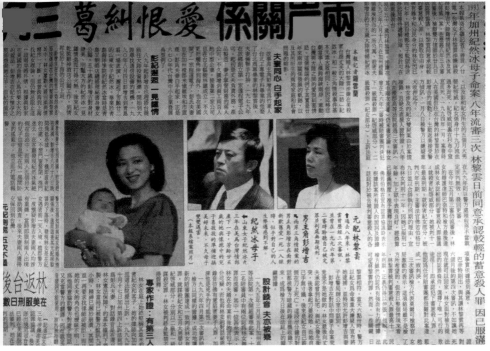

Chinese news article describing the Lisa Peng case.

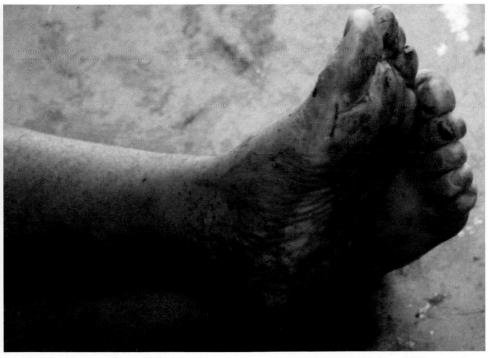

Large amount of medium-velocity blood spatters found on Stephen Haines's feet, which indicates he was standing upright.

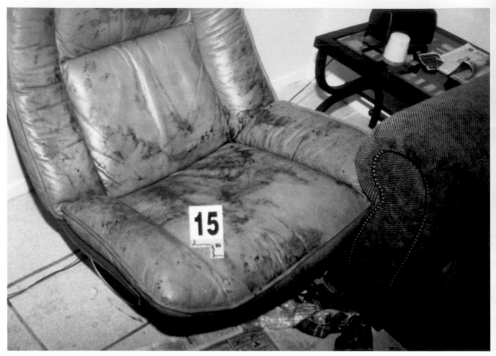

Bloodstain found on the chair in the living room of the Haines-Barratt home.

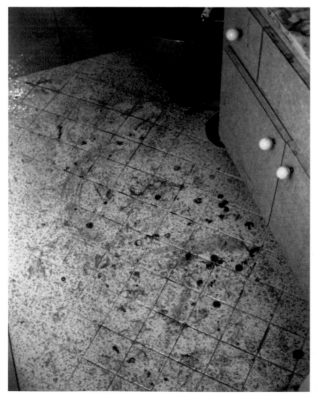

A large amount of blood drops were found on the bathroom floor of the Haines-Barratt home.

friend at a few paces. At the rear of this room there was a small door leading to the wine cellar, which was windowless with brick walls surrounding its bare concrete floor. To get into the room, Ramsey had to pull the door out, toward him. While standing at the door, Ramsey looked to his left and saw a white blanket on the floor, as he was reaching to his right for the room's light switch. Then he turned on the light and saw two hands protruding out from one end of the blanket. Ramsey cried out, "Oh, my God. Oh, my God." He moved forward, with Lucas now behind him, and the two saw JonBenet's body, partially covered by the blanket, her hands extended above her head, apparently tied together. There was masking tape across her mouth. John Ramsey moved forward and pulled the tape from his daughter's mouth and began to take off the binding from one of her wrists. Lucas knelt down and touched one of the little girl's feet and found it cold. Ramsey, after a brief pause, picked up JonBenet's dead body, which was in rigor. Lucas had already bolted upstairs, calling for an ambulance. Ramsey followed up the cellar stairs, holding his dead daughter by her waist, yelling out that JonBenet had been found. Detective Arndt met Ramsey as he emerged and saw the girl's body, with a cord hanging from her right arm, her hands extended over her head, as if posed.

1:05 PM—Arndt ordered Lucas to stand by the head of the basement stairs and not to let anyone go down there. John Ramsey placed his daughter's body on the floor of the front hallway. Arndt saw that the child was dead. Her lips had turned blue, and there was a ligature around her neck, one that had a small, wooden stick attached to it. There was another ligature around her right wrist. She also saw a red circular mark around the base of her throat and a small red heart drawn in ink on her left palm. Patsy Ramsey had remained sitting motionless until Denise Torrell took her by the hand and led her to the front hallway, where Patsy threw herself over her daughter's dead body. She pleaded with Reverend Hoverstock to bring JonBenet back to life. The reverend then led the group in the Lord's Prayer, Patsy sobbing out the words.

1:12 PM—Detective Arndt used a cellular phone to dial 911, and told the dispatcher that JonBenet's body had been found. The dispatcher relayed the news over the police radio that a child's body had been found at the Ramsey house. Arndt next moved JonBenet's body from the hallway, just into the living room, where she laid it at the foot of the Christmas tree. Arndt then paged Larry Mason and the two victim advocates, who had left the home to get lunch.

1:15 PM (approx.)—Sanford Lucas decided to go back down into the basement, wondering why he had not seen JonBenet's body when he had looked around down there earlier that day. He went directly to the wine cellar and, with the light still on, saw the white blanket and a piece of black duct tape lying on it. He felt the tape's stickiness before placing it on the blanket. Looking around the room, he saw it was cluttered by paint cans, window screens, and other supplies. Lucas then went back upstairs. Investigators later found a palm print on the door to the wine cellar, one that they could not identify.

1:20 PM (approx.)—Det. Michael Everett of the Boulder police arrived at the house, as did other uniformed officers. Everett went down into the basement and conducted a thorough search, looking for someone hiding there. In the wine cellar, the detective saw the white blanket and duct tape. He also discovered a child-size, pink nightgown with the word "Barbie" emblazoned on it.

1:25 PM (approx.)—FBI agent Ron Walker and Boulder detective sergeant Larry Mason arrived at the Ramsey house. Both went downstairs and looked at where JonBenet's body had been found. Mason was suspicious about the look of the crime scene. The pair next went to the train room, where they noted the broken window, broken pieces of glass, and a suitcase, set on its side, standing directly under the window, and the scuff marks above the suitcase. Mason then went upstairs, where JonBenet's body was still under the foot of the Christmas tree, and went into action to preserve any portions of the crime scene that had not yet been contaminated. He ordered all nonpolice personnel to vacate the premises.

I think that this minute-by-minute breakdown of events has provided readers with an accessible and essential analysis of the early stages of the investigation. During the seven hours and thirty-three minutes between Patsy Ramsey's initial call and Detective Sergeant Mason's decision to clear the Ramsey house of all nonpolice personnel, a great many things had gone wrong. The most egregious of these errors was the police's failure to discover JonBenet's body, followed closely by John Ramsey's being allowed to move the dead girl's body. These were the direct result of the department's inability to follow proper procedures at the crime scene. The result was many unsupervised adults and officers milling about a crime scene. This entire drama seems like something out of an Agatha Christie novel. Many of the suspects to the crime were in one room, supervised by one detective. And this officer comprehended that she was very overmatched. Yet no backup or other support was forthcoming, even when she called out for help. Besides John Ramsey moving his daughter's body, each time someone touched a surface in the kitchen or any other room, the scene was further contaminated. The large flashlight Officer Weiss saw on the kitchen counter is a perfect example of the point I am making. This potential murder weapon sat on that counter all day long and could have been picked up by any number of persons, all without wearing protective gloves. Finally, late in the day, when no officer had claimed the flashlight, police took it into evidence. A crime scene must be left in its absolute original condition. When found, all evidence has to be properly handled and recorded. There is a vastly better chance that this crime could have been solved, had only these fundamentals to sound police practices been observed.

To get back to what transpired, it's known that Larry Mason planned to get a search warrant and to house the Ramsey family and their friends at a nearby Holiday Inn. He wanted each of JonBenet's parents in a separate room, and he planned to question each independently. Then a policeman overheard John Ramsey talking on the telephone, making flight plans with the pilot of his private plane. When Mason was advised of this, he immediately thought that Ramsey was planning to leave the country. No, Ramsey told Mason, he was planning to take his wife and son to Atlanta, where they had family. Mason told Ramsey that he couldn't do that because they were all needed near the crime scene. Ramsey agreed. Mason felt, at this point, that John Ramsey seemed strangely detached, almost callous. Upon hearing about plans to sequester his family and him at the Holiday Inn, Ramsey balked. He told Mason he wanted to take his family to stay at the Torrells' house. Ramsey appealed for some time before his family and he had to leave their home: "Give us a day." Mason consulted Linda Arndt and then phoned Commander Eller. The consensus was not to push the parents at that time, so Mason relented. A few minutes later, Melinda and John Andrew arrived at the house, driven there from the Denver airport. Both knew about a kidnapping since John Andrew had phoned ahead that morning to his father from the Minneapolis airport. The older children had originally been planning to meet the Ramsey family at the Minneapolis airport later that day, so all six could celebrate the rest of the holidays at their home in Charlevoix, Michigan. John Ramsey then took his older children outside and told them the tragic news of JonBenet's murder. A few minutes later, a patrol car took the four Ramseys to the Torrells' home.

Det. Michael Everett was designated lead investigator on the case, and by 1:50 PM Larry Mason and he had secured the house. The two started preparing their search warrant. By now police investigators had determined that the Ramsey house's exterior bore no marks of a forcible entry, and they also noted there were no foreign footprints left in the estimated five inches of snow around the house, except at its main entryways. Police did find evidence of someone forcing in a back door, but this scarring of the wood was obviously old. The police now decided to split up to press their investigation. Detective Patterson went to the Lucas residence to question Burke Ramsey, where he was told what he had already heard, that the nine-year-old had slept through his mother's finding of the note and the frantic 911 call—that he'd heard nothing unusual overnight. Linda Arndt went to the Torrells' home to continue to question the Ramseys. Just prior to her arrival there, John Ramsey phoned Eugene Stallworth at Access Graphics and tearfully told his personnel director that JonBenet had been found murdered. Stallworth also wept. Boulder police arrived at Stallworth's office an hour later, their second stop there that day. This time the questions seemed much more pointed, and Stallworth, later that evening, told another company vice president, a ten-year veteran, that he'd felt like he was a suspect. The police had specifically asked him about any foreign companies or other foreign parties who might have had a vendetta against Ramsey or Access Graphics. They also wanted to know the names of the company's key players. That night Stallworth made calls from his home to other executives, informing them of Jon-Benet's murder. Some had already heard, and all were horrified. In the next few months as many as thirty employees were questioned by the police, who also searched the hard drives of hundreds of corporate computers.

At police headquarters, Cdr. John Eller was beginning to object to the FBI's continued presence in the case. He felt his department did not need any outside assistance, either from the FBI or from the Colorado Bureau of Investigation. FBI agent Ron Walker had already outlined for Mason the standard procedure for this kind of homicide. Investigators were to question immediate family members first, then domestic employees, and then, others close to the family, such as close friends and business associates. Finally, police should look for outsiders. This procedure, the FBI held, had to be strictly adhered to, and investigators had to be careful not to leapfrog over one of the concentric circles of suspects to get to another. This avoided investigators concentrating too closely on a less-logical suspect, such as a stranger. Eller told Larry Mason that the FBI was no longer needed.

In the middle of the afternoon, Pete Hofstram, who headed the felony division of the Boulder County District Attorney's office, called Bill Wise, the first assistant district attorney, at his home to update him about the finding of JonBenet Ramsey's body. Hofstram had called Wise early in the morning, when he'd first heard about the missing little girl. Wise's boss, District Attorney Alex Hunter, was away in Hawaii on vacation, and Wise decided that things were not pressing enough to call Hunter there. Wise expected a routine call from Hunter before the weekend. Hofstram was frustrated at several aspects of what the police had been doing. His first and foremost frustration was the fact of the police's failure to discover the body earlier that day and their subsequently allowing the crime scene to become so contaminated. But he also complained to Wise about the decision to publicly center their operations at the Ramsey house when the FBI protocol clearly called for the police presence to be off-site, so that the kidnappers could not see their demands about not notifying the authorities were not being met. Marked police cars had been parked outside the Ramsey house since dawn.

Once the police had left the Ramsey house, they could not legally reenter until they had obtained a signed search warrant, a process that took almost six hours. A single officer and an investigator from the coroner's office remained inside standing guard over JonBenet's body. Yellow tape now surrounded the house, and police shivered outside well into the evening, waiting for their reentry. The sparkling Christmas bulbs now eerily provided their light. The ransom note and writing pads that the Ramseys had given police were on their way down to the Colorado Bureau of Investigation. The Ramseys' circle of friends, led by the Lucases and the Torrells, phoned others in their circle to tell them the terrible news. John and Patsy Ramsey picked up their son, Burke, at the Lucases' home and took him to the Torrells', where the three would spend the night. Linda Arndt left the Torrell house, and one officer was stationed there that night to provide security. John Ramsey's corporate attorney and personal friend, Michael Bynum, arrived at the Torrells' house and consoled him. Later that evening, Ramsey and Frank Tor-rell took a walk with Dr. Francesco Beuf, JonBenet's pediatrician, who had arrived with medication for Patsy. When Ramsey returned, he asked Bynum to represent him in the case. Meanwhile, an FBI agent who knew the mother of one of JonBenet's schoolmates called on her, along with a Boulder detective. The FBI agent was specifically interested in whether JonBenet had unexplained absences from school to which the mother said she didn't remember any such problems.

Boulder detectives Patterson and Greg Idler arrived at the home of the housekeeper, Arlene Beckworth. The officers took her hus-band, Fred, downstairs to confine him to his TV room while they questioned his shocked wife upstairs, in their kitchen. Badly shaken, Arlene Beckworth was unable to provide a writing sample for the detectives, since her hands were trembling so severely. She quickly confirmed that Patsy Ramsey had agreed to lend her $2,000 so she could pay her rent. The police questioned her about whether Jon-Benet had ever exhibited any symptoms of sexual molestation and about her bed-wetting habits. Questioned downstairs, Fred Beck-worth said that he'd fallen asleep in front of the TV on Christmas night and had awoken at five the next morning and had gone upstairs where his wife was asleep in their bedroom. The police questioned the couple separately for three hours that night, returned the next day with a warrant and a tape recorder, and closely searched the house and fingerprinted Arlene Beckworth.

In response to questions, Beckworth went back to the day after Thanksgiving, telling police how she and her daughter had searched the Ramsey basement for Christmas decorations, particularly the trees that went into each of the rooms upstairs. They found the missing trees in the small room behind the boiler, where JonBenet's body was later discovered. The basement was also cluttered with Burke's model planes and JonBenet's cowboy boots, hats, and red scarves. Beckworth remembered having a hard time initially opening the door to the train-room, since a recent coat of paint had dried it shut. She also recalled having trouble finding a light switch inside the room, and she did not remember noticing that a window in the room was broken, nor a suitcase or any scuffmarks on the wall below the window. The day after Thanksgiving, Beckworth had her husband, her older married daughter, and her son-in-law distribute the Christmas trees to the rooms upstairs. Since she was not the last person to leave this room, Beckworth did not know if the door to it was left shut. Following her second day of intense questioning, Beckworth wept at her doctor's office as police took strands of her hair and samples of her saliva and blood. Police that day fingerprinted all the members of her family. Meanwhile, Beckworth was left to wonder about how JonBenet had died, since she'd been asked to print the word "beheaded" several times and the police refused to explain why.

Police reentered the Ramsey house at 8:00 PM on December 26 and began their search, focusing on the basement room where Jon-Benet's body had been found as well as the victim's bedroom. At about 8:20 PM, Dr. John Meyer, the Boulder County coroner, accompanied by his top assistant, Patricia Dunn, arrived to find JonBenet's body still under the lighted Christmas tree, now covered by a blanket and a sweatshirt. The pair noted the ligature around Jon-Benet's neck and the one around her right wrist. It was apparent that the cord around the victim's neck had been pulled through a knot, and they saw a broken, varnished piece of wood tied to one end of the cord. Meyer and Dunn also noted a small abrasion on Jon-Benet's right cheek, below her ear. Meyer then left the crime scene, and Dunn stayed on, preparing the body for transport to the morgue. An hour and a half later, Ellen Howard, the seamstress in Longmont, whose daughter, Penny, had coached JonBenet in pageant techniques, was watching the ten o'clock news on television when she saw and heard about the tragedy. Images of JonBenet's public performances were still on the screen when Howard located her daughter, and the two, leaving their holiday guests behind, headed for the Ramsey home, twenty miles away. Once the pair arrived at the lit-up exterior of the partitioned-off Ramsey home, Howard explained to Det. Sgt. Larry Mason their role as close friends of Patsy Ramsey. Mason advised them that he could not give them Mrs. Ramsey's whereabouts, and he asked the mother and daughter to come to see him at police headquarters the next day. The Howards stood there and watched in horror as a gurney carrying a small body bag was taken from the house and placed in the back of an ambulance, which then drove off into the cold December night.

Pete Hofstram, felony division chief at the district attorney's office, appointed Trip DeMuth, a deputy district attorney, to act as a go-between with all of the police investigating the Ramsey case. DeMuth soon reported back to Hofstram that he was very dissatisfied at the minimal amount of evidence collection that the Boulder police seemed to be conducting at the Ramsey house. DeMuth felt that investigators needed to broaden their focus beyond just two locations, the basement room where the body was found and JonBenet's bedroom. He told Hofstram that the police were satisfied that they'd investigated everything after only an hour and a half. Hofstram, hearing this, called Cdr. John Eller and complained. Eller, who had been appointed to his job eleven months earlier, had not yet coordinated a murder investigation in his career, while Hofstram, a fifteen-year veteran as head of the felony division, had worked on twenty-three murders in just the previous four years. Hofstram told Eller that he wanted the house thoroughly searched, including the ripping up of floorboards throughout, and all of it dusted for fingerprints and searched for footprints. The prosecution needed evidence to work with as the case moved to court, he reminded the police commander. Eller immediately saw Hofstram's demands and criticism as a challenge to the police department's control of the investigation. The two purportedly clashed. Rebuffed, Hofstram then took the step of calling Tom Koby, the Boulder police chief, at his home, where he'd been kept abreast of the investigation. Koby got back to Eller and told his commander that he needed to take Hofstram's recommendations more seriously. Ten days later, the Boulder police completed their investigation and turned the home back over to the Ramsey family.

While this battle between Hofstram and Eller erupted, Det. Sgt. Larry Mason stayed at the Ramsey home. At 10:45 that evening, he stepped outside and told a pair of reporters, one from each of Boulder's two daily newspapers, the victim's name and age and then refused to answer questions. Television crews had already left for their 11:00 PM newscasts. Around 11:30, Elliott Zaret, a reporter from the Boulder *Daily Camera*, approached Mason, who initially refused to amplify on his statement. Zaret told Mason that the paper was holding its presses until he filed his story, that the average citizen needed to know more details, and that he had First Amendment rights. After several gruff expletive-laced comments from Mason ("I don't give a fuck about your First Amendment. All I care about is solving this fucking case."), the detective finally agreed to let Zaret print a few facts, including that JonBenet had not been shot or stabbed to death, but Mason would not answer any questions about her possibly being strangled.[9] Zaret's story the next day presented only what Mason had stated. Yet the tension between the Boulder police and the media had also begun. At 11:44 PM, Det. Linda Arndt was the last person to leave the Ramsey home, seventeen and a half hours after she was first paged.

On Friday morning, December 27, shortly after 8:00, Dr. Meyer began his autopsy of JonBenet Ramsey at Boulder Community Hospital. He was assisted by Patricia Dunn, now named Meyer's lead investigator on the case, and Tom Faure. Dets. Linda Arndt and Tom Trujillo of the Boulder police were present, as were Deputy DAs Trip DeMuth and John Pickering, both senior trial litigators. Meyer removed the victim's body from a sealed, white, heavy-plastic bag and took it out of the clean sheet in which it had been wrapped. He also removed paper bags sealed around JonBenet's hands and feet, placed there to preserve potential trace evidence. The experienced coroner, while he gazed down at the clad little body he had seen the previous evening, must have known that in many cases of a child's death, a story about some domestic accident is often created to protect the guilty. Dunn and Trujillo took photos. Dunn eventually shot 113 slides, documenting every stage of the procedure, while Meyer dictated his findings into a tape recorder. He described JonBenet's clothing, including traces of a black fiber, and the cord loosely tied over her nightshirt and around her right wrist. On her right sleeve, Meyer then observed a reddish-brownish stain, about two and a half by one and a half inches in size. This stain was consistent with mucus that could have been wiped from the victim's mouth or nose. The coroner also found urine stains at the crotch and in the front of the long white underpants she wore. On her flowered underpants, which had the word "Wednesday" inscribed on the waistband, he found more urine stains and, at the crotch, three small red spots, each about a half inch in diameter.

Dr. Meyer described the cord around JonBenet's neck: "Wrapped around the neck with a double knot in the midline of the posterior neck is a length of white cord similar to that described as being tied around the right wrist." Meyer then cut through the cord, slipped it off of the body, and finally marked the cord on both sides in case the police wanted to reconstruct the ligature. He was careful not to touch the knot, so the police could study its construction. The knot had two endings of cord, a frayed end four inches long and the other, seventeen inches in length, which ended in several loops tied around a wooden stick that was four and a half inches long. Meyer reported: "This wooden stick is irregularly broken at both ends, and there are several colors of paint and apparent glistening varnish on the surface. Printed in gold letters on one end of the wood [stick] is the word *Korea*." He noted strands of fine blond hair tangled up with the knots in the cord at both ends. He went on: "The white cord is flattened and measures approximately a quarter inch in width. It appears to be made of a white synthetic material. Also secured around the neck is a gold chain with a single charm in the form of a cross." Meyer next described the groove in JonBenet's neck left by the cord. This was almost entirely horizontal, starting in front, just under the bulging caused by the larynx, and circled around the neck to the rear, where the deep red abrasion moved slightly upward. This furrow was close to a half inch in width, with hemorrhaging visible above and below. On the left side of the neck, the groove included a red abrasion, approximately the size of a quarter, a mark Meyer had almost immediately noticed the night before. Meyer and Detective Arndt discussed the dark fibers and a few hairs on the exterior of the victim's nightshirt, which the coroner lifted with forceps and preserved. Also, Meyer noted green strands of a substance mixed into JonBenet's blond hair, something visible to the naked eye. Arndt remembered seeing a likely source for this material: green garlands that had decorated the spiral staircase that led downstairs to the kitchen from JonBenet's room. This completed Dr. Meyer's external examination of the body.

Before the coroner went on to conduct his internal examination of JonBenet's body, Det. Tom Trujillo conducted a final external examination designed to locate any possible semen stains and other deposits. This examination is conducted by passing an ultraviolet (UV) lamp over the surfaces being examined. Trujillo's lamp brought up several traces of black fiber located over the victim's genital area. These were similar to the black traces found on JonBenet's outer garment. Meyer and the detectives also saw a residue on JonBenet's upper thighs that could have been semen. There were other possibilities, though, such as a residue left by other body fluids. The child's underpants had stains that looked like blood, and they also contained the black fiber traces. The corresponding areas of JonBenet's crotch, however, bore no matching blood residue. Meyer told the two detectives that the blood traces and the fibers found in the victim's vaginal area indicated that those surfaces had been wiped clean by someone using a clothlike substance.

With this last external testing completed, Meyer then proceeded with his internal examination. On JonBenet's skull, he discovered a linear fracture on the right side, one that had not been visible to him until he had cut into the skull. This fracture ran approximately eight and a half inches from the front of her head to above her right ear. Toward the back of her head, at the end of this fracture, he also found a displaced rectangular section of the skull, approximately three quarters by a half inch in length. He concluded that a very heavy blow had caused this severe trauma to JonBenet's skull. Moving on, Meyer found small amounts of semidried and dried blood at the entrance to the victim's vagina and a reddening in the vaginal walls. This was heaviest on the right side, from an exterior point of view, and toward the rear of the cavity. The hymen did not show fresh damage, but it had only a rim of tissue running from the upper left at about ten o'clock, to the two o'clock position. Additionally, Meyer found an abrasion on the hymen's orifice at its lower left-hand quadrant, the seven o'clock position. While he conducted his examination of JonBenet's genital area, Dr. Meyer told Detectives Arndt and Trujillo that, in his opinion, the victim could have suffered vaginal penetration, consistent with a sexual assault. Meyer concluded his autopsy at 2:20 PM.

At about ten on the morning of the autopsy, Sanford Lucas, John Ramsey's best friend, arrived at the Boulder police headquarters, where Dets. Fred Patterson and Greg Idler interviewed him. Lucas described how he'd hosted a Christmas dinner party later in the day for the four Ramseys, as well as other family and friends. The next morning, one of his guests was awakened by a call at around 6:00 AM, and his wife, Renee, was soon getting the terrible news of JonBenet's kidnapping from a hysterical Patsy Ramsey. Lucas and Renee hurried over to their friends' home. The police and Frank Torrell were already in the house. A short while after his arrival, Lucas decided to go down into the basement to search for JonBenet. There he found some lights on, and he began calling out the little girl's name. Since the basement was extremely cluttered, he had difficulty moving about, even with lighting. He began looking into the side rooms off of the basement's main boiler chamber, starting with Burke Ramsey's train room. There he saw a suitcase (owned by John Andrew Ramsey, John Ramsey's son, it was later determined) sitting upright on its side under a broken window. Below the window he found shards of the broken glass on the room's concrete floor, some of which he placed on the windowsill. Lucas then moved the suitcase aside, so he could take a closer look at the broken window, noting that its frame was closed but not latched. Leaving the train room, he moved to his right in the boiler room. At the back of the room, behind the boiler, he approached a single, closed-off room that John and Patsy had referred to as their "wine cellar." The door had a closed wooden latch that Lucas turned, so he could open the door. He didn't enter the room, which was pitch-black. He tried to find a light switch, and, when he couldn't locate one, he closed the door and continued his basement search. He told the detectives that he could not remember if he had relatched the door. Then he returned upstairs. Later on, Lucas told his friend Frank Torrell about the broken window. The two detectives pressed Lucas on why he had not seen JonBenet's body when he stood at the door to the chamber where she was later found by her father, and Lucas had no answer.

Sanford Lucas continued on with his narrative on what he had seen and done the day before. At three in the afternoon, upon John Ramsey's request, Lucas had called John Ramsey's pilot to cancel the flight to Atlanta that Ramsey had scheduled. Lucas later went to his own home and told his two children about JonBenet's death. In the evening, Lucas stopped by the Torrells' home, where his wife had already gone, on his way to Denver International Airport to meet Jeff Ramsey, John's Brother, and Hugh Averill, Ramsey's financier. John Ramsey volunteered to go with Lucas, and the four returned to the Torrell home by 11 PM, that night. Lucas's interview had lasted the better part of that morning.

Cdr. John Eller met with the media early in the afternoon of Friday, December 27, in a first-floor conference room in Boulder's Public Safety Building. Earlier that day many of the reporters from the local papers and television channels had fanned out in the University Hill neighborhood, asking questions about the Ramseys and JonBenet. One newsman knew Reverend Hoverstock and was very familiar with St. John's Episcopal Church. Yet, like the others, he found that the people who knew the Ramseys best were very tight-lipped, saying only that the family had been in Boulder since 1991 and were very nice. All those questioned were, quite naturally, shocked over the murder of JonBenet. Their answers also focused on the Ramsey family's status and their owning a vacation home in Michigan and the other amenities that go along with great success. During his first meeting with the press, Commander Eller seemed uncomfortable and was very guarded in the information he put out. Over his shoulder, reporters and photographers saw a photo of a smiling JonBenet Ramsey on a bulletin board. Eller confirmed the fact that the victim's body had been discovered by a family member, but did not identify John Ramsey. He said, her "death was clearly the result of a criminal act." Eller explained that the police failure to find the body was a consequence of their initial belief that they were dealing with a kidnapping. He said that the Ramsey family was staying with friends, they were "going through a tremendous grieving process," and that a police officer was on those premises for "security" purposes. He added that the parents were going to be interviewed and then referred to the family as "well-connected with Boulder society." The reporters asked Eller about the ransom note, and the commander gave this perplexing answer: "The ransom note was a typical—if there is such a thing—kidnapping ransom note, the kind you'd find in any movie." Eller did not rule out the possibility that JonBenet had been murdered during a "bona fide" kidnapping attempt. "We have no reason to believe that it was [a kidnapping] or not at this time." Then, he added, "It's too early in the investigation to start ruling things out." When questioned further about the note, Eller said that it demanded money and also mentioned "future demands."

After Sanford Lucas had completed his interview around noon, he dropped by the Torrells' home to console John and Patsy Ramsey and be with the others at the house. About four, Lucas left and went to the office of Michael Bynum, John Ramsey's corporate attorney, to fill him in on the situation. At Access Graphics's headquarters, Eugene Stallworth was very hard at work, initially meeting with an executive committee to advise the company's leadership of what had happened and how to handle the situation. One participant predicted that, with JonBenet's status as a beauty queen, her death was going to take on global proportions in the news media. All agreed that the business and this personal tragedy were to be kept separate. Stallworth even wondered whether the press release he'd insisted be put out earlier in the month on Access Graphics's recently passing the $1 billion barrier in sales had helped cause the tragedy. Did this story, which included a photo of John Ramsey, cause the family to be targeted? Rather than agonize over thoughts like that, the group established reporting procedures on major developments in the investigation and ways to inform others who were away on Christmas breaks. Stallworth was also in close touch with Lockheed Martin's key executives to determine what was going to be done in light of John Ramsey's absence and out of respect for his going through a grieving process. A select group of Access Graphics managers were to report directly to Gary Mann at Lockheed Martin for the next three months. Otherwise, Lockheed Martin had complete confidence in the management team that John Ramsey had assembled. Business was to be carried on as usual.

Following the news conference, John Eller met with Detectives Arndt and Trujillo to discuss the autopsy's results. Earlier in the day, Eller had assigned thirty officers to the case, almost one-third of the one hundred or so on the force. Det. Sgt. Larry Mason was named to head the daily assignments. Mason, whose family went back four generations in Colorado, a rarity, came from a public service background. This included his father, who had spent a career as a member of the Boulder fire department and an uncle who been with the sheriff's department for thirty years. Mason and Eller, however, continued to clash on the way the case was being run, which became a growing problem. As Eller sat down to listen to what Linda Arndt and Tom Trujillo had to report, he must have been very conscious of the statistical fact that a substantial percentage of child murders were committed by the father. Eller also knew that there was no evidence of a forced entry into the Ramsey house. He knew that John Ramsey had already told Sanford Lucas that months earlier he had broken the window in the train room, when he'd found himself locked out of the house. Investigators had also found an intact spider web woven in an iron grating over the well outside the basement window, one that would surely have been broken if someone had recently climbed down to get in or out of the basement window. By now, the Colorado Bureau of Investigation (CBI) had preliminarily reported back on the ransom note, stating that the paper for the note had come from one of the white, lined pads given to police by John Ramsey. The CBI also reported that their investigators had established that the actual ransom note had been preceded by the drafting of a practice note by someone using the same pad. All of this, added to the autopsy's evidence of a possible sexual assault, meant, Eller said, that JonBenet's parents had to be interviewed as soon as possible. John and Patsy were now prime suspects, particularly the father. After Eller's meeting with Arndt and Trujillo, Eller ordered that John Ramsey's office at Access

Graphics be sealed and that an officer be posted as a guard until a legal search could be completed.

Later that evening, Detective Sergeant Mason and Detective Arndt went to the Torrells' home to interview John and Patsy Ramsey. However, Patsy was still in very bad shape, crying constantly and under heavy medication. Bordering on the clinical definition of shock, Mrs. Ramsey could not be cogently interviewed. The two detectives turned their attention to John Ramsey, who agreed to sit down with them in the Torrells' living room. Flanked by Jeff Ramsey, his brother, and Hugh Averill, his broker and friend, Ramsey mumbled out a few sentences to each of the questions the detectives asked. Michael Bynum, his corporate attorney, sat at a far end of the room, but within hearing distance. Mason realized that his best move was to schedule interviews in the next day or so, rather than persist. He had already underscored for the Ramseys the critical importance that their promptly answering police questions would play in finding their child's murderer. John Ramsey told the detectives he could not yet commit to a time for his wife and him to answer their questions. John Ramsey stayed up until 2:00 the following morning, sobbing and being consoled by his friends. Late that same night, Dr. Meyer, accompanied by Dr. Andrew Sirotnak, assistant professor of pediatrics at Colorado University's Health Sciences Center, reexamined JonBenet Ramsey's body for sexual assault, and the two agreed that there had been an injury to her vagina.

The next morning, Saturday, December 28, dawned brightly in Boulder, with blue skies and an unusually beautiful view of the Rocky Mountains in one direction and of the Continental Divide in another. Attorney Michael Bynum awoke with an equally clear insight on what he should now recommend to his friend and business client, John Ramsey: get the best criminal attorney available and stop giving any more statements to the police. Bynum himself had briefly worked as a deputy district attorney in Boulder, before going into business transactions and overall corporate law. Without consulting either John or Patsy Ramsey, Bynum called the Boulder police and told them that the Ramseys were not going to give any more testimony to the police, especially privileged information, without their criminal lawyer being present. Bynum then called attorney Bryan Morgan of the top-flight Denver firm Haddon, Morgan and Foreman; by nightfall the Ramseys had retained Morgan. Linda Arndt, hearing about these developments, called Pete Hofstram of the district attorney's office for help. Hofstram called Bynum, who confirmed that the Ramseys refused any more interviews, yet Bynum agreed that all members of the family, including John Andrew and Melinda, would provide hair, saliva, fingerprint, blood, and handwriting samples. Bynum also agreed to detectives interviewing John Andrew, Melinda, and John Ramsey's brother, Jeff, who were all now at the Torrells' house.

When he heard about this turn of events, John Eller became angry and frustrated. While Pete Hofstram was setting up a schedule with Michael Bynum for the Ramsey family to provide the blood and other samples, he was interrupted by a call from Eller. The police commander told Hofstram that he'd learned that John and Patsy planned to leave for Atlanta within a day or so to bury their daughter there. Eller demanded formal police interviews before this departure, or else. He planned to refuse the release of JonBenet's remains until those interviews were completed. Hofstram was shocked at this strategy and bluntly told Eller that what he planned was not legal.[10] The commander, apparently, wanted to rectify the mistakes made by his police during the first few days of the investigation. Eller did not waver, and the conversation ended on that sour note. After he'd hung up his phone, Eller told Larry Mason about his strategy. The detective was also incredulous and advised Eller that what he planned would violate the Ramsey family's rights.[11] Mason sensed that a bad situation was rapidly deteriorating. Finally, Dr. Meyer, the coroner, refused to cooperate with Eller's plan, and, since his autopsy was completed, he agreed to release JonBenet's body to the child's family. Michael Bynum did not tell either Patsy or John Ramsey what Eller had been threatening. Much later on that Saturday, Boulder district attorney Alex Hunter called his top assistant, Bill Wise, and was told about Eller's aborted attempt to withhold the victim's body. Hunter quickly joined the chorus of disapproval.

Late that Saturday afternoon, John and Patsy Ramsey arrived at the Boulder Justice Center, which housed the sheriff's, district attorney's, and coroner's offices, as well as the courts, where they provided more samples of their handwriting. Patsy was heavily sedated and, at times, seemed to be on the verge of collapse. Besides her handwriting samples, police asked Mrs. Ramsey to reprint some of the text of the ransom note, and Patsy wasn't able to comply. Melinda Ramsey also went there for her first interview with police. Det. Kim Stewart questioned Melinda for more than two hours. Police were particularly interested in how she and her brother, John Andrew, spent the critical hours of Christmas evening until dawn the next morning. In Melinda's case, she told the detectives that she'd gotten off her nursing shift at a hospital in Marietta, Georgia, at seven on Christmas morning and had gone to the home of her mother, Lucinda Johnson, where John Andrew was staying. Later that day, John Andrew, Melinda, her boyfriend, Lucinda Johnson, and her friend Elliot Whitmore* all gathered there, where they exchanged Christmas gifts. As the afternoon wore on, the entire party went across the street to a neighbor's home, where they had Christmas dinner. After that, Melinda and her boyfriend went home to pack for her early-morning flight to Minneapolis, where she and her brother planned to meet their dad and his family. About 9:00 PM, Melinda and her boyfriend went to visit her boyfriend's uncle at his home, and they were back home by midnight.

Dets. Ron Gosage and Steve Thomas questioned John Andrew for two hours, starting at 6:00 that evening. John Andrew had gone to a Christmas service on Christmas Eve with Lucinda Johnson and Elliot Whitmore at the Peachtree Presbyterian Church in Atlanta. He had spent the earlier portion of Christmas day at home with his mother and Elliot and then had been part of the family gathering that Melinda had also described. Later on Christmas evening, at about 8:30, John Andrew had gone to a friend's home in Marietta to play video games. An hour later he was picked up by another friend to see a 10:30 PM movie at the Town and Country Movie Theaters in Marietta. After the movie he had been taken back to the original friend's house to get his car and was home at his mother's by 1:00

AM. The next morning Melinda picked John Andrew up, and they made their 8:36 AM flight to Minneapolis, where the entire Ramsey clan had planned to leave for their Michigan vacation. Later on, Boulder police detectives went over John Andrew's account of his whereabouts, factoring in the possibility that one or more of his friends could possibly be lying to provide him with an alibi. Even with that possibility, John Andrew would have only had a six- or seven-hour window of opportunity to catch a flight to Denver, drive to Boulder, enter the house, kill JonBenet, and then catch a flight back to Atlanta, where he'd been seen early the next morning. The police also combed the records of all the airlines flying between Atlanta and Denver that evening and did not find any record of John Andrew's making those round-trip flights. This investigation effectively eliminated both Melinda and John Andrew as suspects in the killing of their younger half sister.

On Sunday morning, December 29, a memorial service was held for JonBenet Ramsey at St. John's Episcopal Church in Boulder. Dets. Linda Arndt, Steve Thomas, and Ron Gosage and Det. Sgt. Larry Mason all attended. Other officers also videotaped all of the participants. This was standard operating procedure, since the police were alert to the possibility of a felon revisiting either the scene of a crime or some other critical location or occasion, such as this service. John Ramsey spoke about his daughter and wore a medallion that Jon-Benet had won in the achievement portion of one of her pageants. This, he had told his daughter, was due to intelligence and not to just her appearance. Patsy Ramsey's two sisters, Pam and Polly, were also in attendance, as were many of the couple's closest friends. The entire service lasted a little under an hour. The Reverend Rol Hoverstock prayed that the little girl's murderer would be quickly found, especially since so many people in Boulder now were worried about a killer being in the area. After the service, Patsy Ramsey was helped up the aisle by her husband, and she stopped to embrace some of her friends there. John kept repeating to her, "I need you to be strong." Outside, the national and international media were attempting to swarm in on the family. By now the press included in its ranks the tabloids with their troublesome photographers.

Boulder police detective Steve Thomas helped the Ramseys to their waiting car. Later that day, the family left for the Jefferson County Airport near Boulder for a flight to Atlanta on a Lockheed Martin corporate jet. After nightfall, a Delta flight took off out of Denver and carried JonBenet's body to Atlanta. After the services at St. John's Church, the rest of the mourners were invited to a quiet reception in the parish hall.

At least two of the participants at the service were suspects. Arlene Beckworth, the Ramseys' housekeeper, embraced Patsy's sister, Pam, who redirected her over to Patsy. The two consoled one another, and Arlene quietly asked her former boss about whether all of the exterior entrances to the house had been locked that night. Patsy Ramsey assured Arlene that all the locks had been put in place. Then Patsy was in the arms of another friend. This was the last time that Arlene ever saw or talked to either John or Patsy Ramsey. Another suspect was Austin O'Rourke, the older gentleman who had been Santa Claus at the Ramseys' Christmas party on the evening of December 23. He was possibly the source, therefore, of the promise of a late-night Christmas visit to JonBenet for the presentation of a special present, the Santa Claus promise that JonBenet had told her playmate about on the morning of Christmas Eve, a declaration that the playmate's mother had then clarified with JonBenet. O'Rourke, as noted, was a retired professor of journalism at Colorado University and had worked for the Ramseys often enough that they'd given him a key to their home. Also, police detectives discovered that O'Rourke did not have a real alibi for his whereabouts on Christmas night. He had, he told the police, slept at home that night, a report his wife corroborated. O'Rourke was also asked to speak at the service, but his rambling and seemingly incoherent remarks made several of the mourners uncomfortable.

Late that Sunday afternoon, Det. Linda Arndt faxed a two-page memo containing sixteen questions for the Ramseys to Bryan Morgan, the Denver attorney who first represented John Ramsey. In a preamble to the questions, Arndt noted that John, Patsy, and Burke Ramsey were out of town and nobody yet knew when they would return to Boulder to be interviewed. The first four of these questions centered on the time each went to bed and to sleep, whether their bedroom doors were open or closed, and whether there were any radios or television sets left on that could cover any noise. The fifth question asked if JonBenet had eaten shortly before she went to bed. This was a particularly significant query since Arndt knew that the coroner had found five partially digested pineapple chunks in Jon-Benet's stomach. The next three questions related to Patsy Ramsey's finding the ransom note, what she did next, and whom she first contacted after she discovered it. Then Arndt asked about how John Ramsey found out that his daughter was missing. The next three questions inquired about the interior and exterior lighting of the house and who had checked that the doors were locked and whether other access points were all secure. The thirteenth question asked what JonBenet had been wearing when she went to bed. The next two questions asked what the family's plans were for the next morning and what time each woke up the next day. The last question asked if any of the three had gotten up during the night. Arndt's questions were an obvious response to a situation that was now deeply bothering the detectives working the case: key witnesses had not ever been interviewed and now these three had traveled out of the jurisdiction, thousands of miles away, and nobody knew when or if they would return, let alone be interviewed. Linda Arndt had also received a request from Sanford Lucas, John Ramsey's close friend, to go into the home and retrieve a kitten doll of JonBenet's, so she could be buried with this favorite toy. The day before, a member of the family had been allowed to take out other special belongings. Arndt did as asked and gave the kitten to Renee Lucas, who took the stuffed doll to Atlanta when she and her husband flew there for the funeral the next day.

On that Monday, Linda Arndt reinterviewed Sanford Lucas, a day before he and his wife left for Atlanta. Lucas was convinced that someone with some kind of grudge against the Ramsey family had broken into their home and killed JonBenet. Lucas even suggested that the parent of one of JonBenet's pageant competitors might have struck back at the little girl for some perceived wrong. A couple of hours after this interview, Arndt and Det. Jane Harmer again met with Lucas, along with Frank Torrell, at the latter's Boulder office. Both Lucas and Torrell told the two detectives that they were worried that John Ramsey's older son, John Andrew Ramsey, had become a suspect, and they both vouched for the twenty-year-old. Within an hour of this second interview, the Lucases and the Torrells left for the Denver airport.

Linda Arndt promptly reported back to Cdr. John Eller about the family's friends' concerns over John Andrew, and she suggested that, at the press briefing scheduled for later that day, police could put out the word that the two older siblings had been cleared as suspects. Eller was receptive. At their briefing, police specified for the media that both John Andrew and Melinda had been established as out of state the night of the murder, but neither sibling had been entirely cleared as a suspect. Arndt then called the Ramseys in Atlanta and told them of this declaration. At this point, it is very interesting to note that Linda Arndt met with Commander Eller after she had faxed her sixteen questions to John Ramsey's defense lawyer. Later on, Detective Arndt would be excoriated for sending that fax. Both her peers on the force and several of the prosecuting attorneys felt that she should never have taken that step on her own. This very transmission violated an ancient police interrogation belief: never tip your hand on what you will be asking a suspect, and always preserve the element of surprise so you can use it to its fullest advantage. They felt that the faxed questions to a defense attorney, in particular, played into the Ramseys' hands. Any and all answers could be sifted through their lawyers' hands. This screening even gave the Ramseys a chance to anticipate follow-up questions, another major weapon in a bright and dedicated interrogator's arsenal. But did Arndt discuss this fax with John Eller in their meeting? Had she even discussed and reviewed the questions with Eller ahead of time and later simply took the rap for their combined decision? Eller's principal strength in the Boulder Police Department was the loyalty many in its ranks held for him. Like so many other aspects of this case, there is a solid chance that no one will ever be able to clarify the events that led to Linda Arndt's faxing those sixteen questions to the Ramseys' attorney.

The following Monday afternoon, Assistant District Attorney Pete Hofstram received a letter from Bryan Morgan, John Ramsey's recently retained defense lawyer. Morgan wanted to be advised prior to any forensic evidence in the case being tested in a way that might destroy that evidence. He also wanted to grant prior approval for any forensic testing on evidence voluntarily provided by the Ramseys. He then asked for the return of any and all keys to the Ramsey home given to the police by the couple and a copy of the ransom note, the affidavits for the two search warrants, and the autopsy report. With District Attorney Alex Hunter away on vacation, top assistant Bill Wise and Hofstram were in charge of the case's investigation. At about the same time, Boulder County sheriff George Epp was meeting with several of his top deputies, who criticized the way John Eller was handling the case. Some Boulder police detectives seemed to be just sitting around, when they could have been out gathering statements and looking for evidence.[12] On the day the child's body was found, Epp had lent the Boulder police three of his detectives to assist the undermanned department. This help was no longer needed, it seemed. Sheriff Epp called Boulder police chief Tom Koby and said several of his people wanted to help, but Koby refused this offer. A blue wall was going up around the Boulder Police Department. This was their case, and they alone were going to solve it.

On Monday afternoon, December 30, JonBenet Ramsey's body lay in an open casket at the Mayes-Ward-Dobbins Funeral Home in Marietta, Georgia. Hundreds of mourners filed by, paying their respects to the Ramsey family and to the little girl, who lay with a pageant crown on her blonde head. The next morning, New Year's Eve, JonBenet's remains were moved to the Peachtree Presbyterian Church in Atlanta for her funeral. A few hours before dawn, prior to the body's being moved, the Boulder police had contacted the Marietta force and asked their detectives to take tracings of and measures of JonBenet's hands and feet. After the body was moved to Atlanta, hundreds of additional mourners passed by the casket. The Reverend Frank Harrington, who had married JonBenet's parents in that same church sixteen years earlier and had later baptized their only daughter, conducted the services. In his homily, Reverend Harrington said, "The mind cannot accept, and the heart refuses to grasp, the death of one so young, who is suddenly taken from us by the cruelty and malice of some unworthy person." He added to the thousand or so who packed the church, "When a child is lost, one feels part of the future is gone." The funeral cortege then traveled to Marietta, to St. James Episcopal Cemetery, where JonBenet was buried.

John and Patsy Ramsey, along with Burke, were staying at her parents', Don and Nedra Paugh's, home in nearby Roswell. The day before the funeral, Gary Mann, Ramsey's Access Graphics liaison with Lockheed Martin, had visited John at the Paughs' home, and he stayed with John Ramsey until early the next morning. After the funeral, the family and their best friends retired to the Paugh residence. During the course of the afternoon, a very bitter and loud argument broke out between John Ramsey and his best friend, Sanford Lucas. With Patsy nervously standing by, Lucas confronted Ramsey about his hiring a defense lawyer and the couple's avoiding police interviews. Lucas had heard that Ramsey was planning to hire his own investigative team, and this was absolutely the wrong direction for him to take, Sanford Lucas loudly told Ramsey. Lucas had also gotten wind of the Ramseys' calling the CNN meganews network, based in Atlanta, for an interview. His daughter had just been buried, Lucas barked at a now red-faced Ramsey. He should be headed back to Boulder to help the police there find JonBenet's murderer. At the end of his tirade, Lucas had his hands up close to John Ramsey's face. Along with John Ramsey, the entire room had fallen dead silent. Lucas finally broke off his torrent of words, and the two men separated, no longer friends of any kind. John Ramsey wasn't the only person present who'd become very uncomfortable over Lucas's very uncharacteristic behaviors. Frank Torrell was aghast at what had happened and at Lucas's behavior.[13]

What Sanford Lucas had been hearing about CNN proved to be accurate. Brian Cabell, a CNN correspondent who on New Year's Eve morning had been outside JonBenet's funeral at the Peachtree Presbyterian Church in Atlanta, was quietly celebrating the coming of the new year at home with his family when he received a call from the president of CNN, Tom Johnson. Earlier that day, executives at

CNN had heard from friends of John and Patsy Ramsey that the couple wanted to go on national television as soon as possible to clear the air on why they hadn't seemed fully cooperative with the Boulder police and to dispel some rumors implicating them in their daughter's death. They also wanted to address the question of why they appeared to be avoiding the media. Cabell scheduled the interview, one he was most eager to conduct, since this provided CNN with an important scoop, for later the next morning, New Year's Day. At midmorning on New Year's Day, Cabell took a cab out to the Paughs' home in Roswell, a step to protect the Ramseys' privacy, and rode back to CNN with the couple, along with Jeff Ramsey. Cabell also wanted to use the forty-minute cab ride as a time to get to know the Ramseys, a kind of preinterview. He saw that Patsy Ramsey appeared as though she had been crying for several days and that John Ramsey was impassive. On the way into town, the Ramseys directly answered most of Cabell's questions, though Jeff jumped in several times to answer for his brother. Otherwise, there were long periods of silence during the trip.

Once the couple was settled in front of cameras in a sixth-floor conference room at CNN headquarters, Cabell started the taped interview by asking why the couple had chosen that particular time and place to speak out. He also noted that John and Patsy seemed to have pulled together as a team. John answered the first question by saying that he and his wife had felt "pretty isolated" and he wanted to thank all of the individuals who cared about them. He then added, "For our grief to resolve itself, we now have to find out why this happened." A few moments later, Cabell asked John Ramsey how he'd found JonBenet's body, and the father said that Sanford Lucas and he had been asked to go into the basement, and Ramsey had then found the body, adding that "there were no windows in that room." As the questions moved forward, John Ramsey interjected answers for his wife and quietly took control of their dialogue. Then Cabell asked why the family had retained a lawyer, prefixing this with the comment that "most laymen" would not understand that move. John Ramsey responded that, besides a lawyer, he was also assembling his own "investigative team. I want the best minds this country has to offer to help us to resolve this."

Cabell next directly asked Mrs. Ramsey about finding the ransom note. She recounted how she had just awoken and she'd descended the back stairs, as usual, heading for the kitchen. She said she had seen the pieces of paper in the dim light, spread across the runner of one of the stairs, and told how she had seen that it was a note addressed to her husband. Patsy Ramsey quoted the note: " 'We have your daughter.' It just wasn't registering. I don't know if I got farther than that, and I immediately ran back upstairs and I pushed open her [JonBenet's] door and she was not in her bed and I screamed for John." John Ramsey then interjected how he'd scanned the note, especially about not calling the authorities and how he'd immediately directed his wife to call the police. Patsy continued: "We were just frantic, and I immediately dialed the police, 911, and [the operator] was trying to calm me down and I said our child had just been kidnapped. I was just screaming. 'Send help. Send help.' I dialed some of my very closest friends. 'Come quickly.' [Then] an officer was there. It seems like an eternity, but I know it was just minutes." Cabell then asked Patsy Ramsey whether the police had questioned her husband and her, and Mrs. Ramsey gave the answer that began this chapter. Cabell later repeated her ending words, "There is a killer on the loose," toward the end of the interview. He pointed out that the police had denied this, and he asked if Mrs. Ramsey thought that the assailant had come from outside her home. Patsy Ramsey then repeated, "There is a killer on the loose," and John Ramsey injected, "Absolutely." Patsy then added, "I don't know who, if it's a he or a she. . . . But if I was a resident of Boulder, I would tell my friends to keep . . ." and she began to cry at this point. John Ramsey consoled his wife with the words "It's OK." Mrs. Ramsey was then able to add, "Keep your babies close to you. There's someone out there."

As he began to conclude the interview, Cabell began to frame his next question with the comment "Speculation on talk shows will focus on you . . . " and John Ramsey cut him off with the comment "It's nauseating beyond belief." Patsy Ramsey then added, "America has just been hurt so deeply with this—the tragic things that have happened." She alluded to the 1996 South Carolina case where a mother, Susan Smith, had drowned her two children by driving her car into a pond. Mrs. Ramsey then cited the O. J. Simpson case. She concluded her comments with: "America is suffering because [it has] lost faith in the American family. . . . She'll [JonBenet] never have to know the loss of a child. She will never have to know cancer or the death of a child." John Ramsey then added: "We learned when we lost our first child that people would come forward to us and that sooner or later, everyone carries a very heavy burden in this life. And JonBenet didn't carry any burdens." The interview completed, the Ramseys took a cab back out to Roswell. Later on that afternoon, when the well-promoted interview first aired nationally, Cabell reported that John Ramsey had also confirmed for him the fact that his daughter's mouth had been covered over by duct tape when he first found her. He also noted that Mr. Ramsey did not remember seeing a cord around JonBenet's neck, concluding that he possibly had panicked when he picked up her body, in his haste to get her upstairs where she might be brought back to life.

The Ramseys' CNN interview took up half of the network's evening newscast and got very wide viewership around the country. In the Boulder area, the newscast landed like a bombshell. The local CNN outlet in Denver put Brian Cabell on the air live and asked why the couple had chosen to speak to him, and out of Atlanta, since Cabell had not yet covered the case. Cabell had no answer. There is no public record of the Boulder police response to this extraordinary step by the Ramseys, but the irony that a relative stranger to the case, a newsman in Atlanta, was able to ask JonBenet's parents a series of probing questions while they could not, this could not have been lost on them.

Back in Boulder, the police had been very active, screening the Ramseys' neighborhood and asking questions of Access Graphics employees. John Ramsey's executive secretary told investigators about Todd Ogilvy, a former Access Graphics employee who Ramsey himself had mentioned to police on December 26 as a person who had a grudge against him. Ogilvy and Ramsey had first met in 1971 when the two worked together for AT&T in Ohio. In 1994 Ramsey had hired Ogilvy for Access Graphics, but the old friend did not seem to fit into his new environment. Ramsey then moved Ogilvy into a post as director of security. With the acquisition by Lockheed Martin, Ramsey found that he could no longer justify Ogilvy's six-figure salary and had to demote him. Rather than take this cut in pay, Ogilvy left Access Graphics, claiming that the company owed him $118,000, the exact figure later demanded in the ransom note. Ogilvy eventually settled with the company for half of that amount. Ogilvy, it was also discovered, had made a statement threatening revenge on John Ramsey, one that was overheard by a member of the corporation's board of directors.[14] Upon his departure, Ogilvy had sent a lengthy fax to Lockheed Martin denouncing Ramsey, particularly the way he dealt with his employees. On December 31, Dets. Fred Patterson and Carey Weinheimer interviewed Ogilvy at his home in Louisville, which was fifteen minutes from the Ramseys' neighborhood. Ogilvy said that his wife and he had spent Christmas afternoon and evening visiting with family and friends, returning home by 8:00 PM. The two had retired early since Mrs. Ogilvy was not feeling well. The next morning, December 26, Ogilvy left his home for his new job in Littleton by 6:30 AM. Since the husband and wife were the only means for establishing an alibi for one another, Todd Ogilvy remained an active suspect.

Working door to door in the Ramseys' upscale University Hill neighborhood, police looked for any fact or unusual circumstance that had occurred on the evening of December 25 to the early morning of December 26. One Ramsey neighbor told investigators that around midnight he'd looked out his window and had seen a light shining in the Ramseys' kitchen. At another house, one said he hadn't noticed anything strange about the Ramsey house as he looked out his window at the home, watching late-night television. Another neighbor told Det. Barry Hartkopp that she had looked over at the Ramseys' house that night and had noted that a safety light on the southeast corner of the house was not on, something she'd found unusual since that light had illuminated that area for years. Then there was the lady, whose bedroom window was partially open that night, who was certain she'd heard a horrifying scream from the Ramsey house a short while after midnight. This sound was so loud, she said, that it surely must have awoken the Ramseys. Another neighbor said that at 8:00 the next morning he'd noticed a side door to the Ramsey house had been left open. By that time, though, police reasoned, many people had already been in or around the house, any one of whom could have left that door ajar. That morning, Boulder officer Larry Burton had found a small earring on the curb in front of the Ramseys' house. Unclaimed, this, too, could have come from anyone.

Detectives interviewed an elderly couple who lived directly across the street from the Ramseys and who had been given a key to the house, since they often looked after JonBenet's dog, a bichon frise named Jacques. In preparation for the Ramsey family's departure for Michigan, Jacques was already in their home the night of the murder. The couple had been guests at the Ramseys' December 23 Christmas party. The gentleman was seventy-seven and suffered from palsy so severe that he could not provide a handwriting sample. Later, a doctor's note confirmed that condition. Just before the holiday, John Ramsey had used their house to stash a bicycle that he later gave JonBenet on Christmas morning. This couple also had a boarder who came under suspicion, a man who had also attended the Ramseys' Christmas party, but had not met either Patsy or Jon-Benet. This individual had been suffering from stomach flu on Christmas evening and said he'd stayed home that evening, watching television in the den upstairs with his landlords before retiring to his basement apartment. Det. Steve Thomas obtained handwriting samples and fingerprinted this man. Later, this individual took and passed a lie detector test.

Cdr. John Eller certainly noticed the Ramseys' CNN interview. Instead of their being in deep shock, the Ramseys seemed quite able to discuss the case. Eller decided to dispatch Det. Sgt. Larry Mason, and Dets. Steve Thomas, Tom Trujillo, Ron Gosage, and Jane Harmer to Atlanta to check alibis and to conduct background checks on the Ramseys and their friends. The police had already been tipped off on Sanford Lucas's highly vocal attack on John Ramsey at the Paughs' residence, so Lucas became an early call for Trujillo and Harmer. They questioned Lucas and his wife, Renee, in

their hotel room at 8:30 on the morning of January 2. Lucas confirmed the altercation he'd had with Ramsey, one that got so
intense that Don Paugh, Patsy's father, had felt it necessary to inter-
vene. Lucas and his wife were now planning to return to Boulder on
an afternoon flight. The rift between Ramsey and him had become
irreparable. Looking back at the chaotic events of a week earlier,
Lucas now was wondering why he, on December 26, had not been
able to find JonBenet's body in the wine cellar when he'd conducted at midmorning his sole search of the basement. He had
actually opened the door to the darkened, windowless room where
the little body lay, yet had not spotted the white blanket. And, back
in Boulder, the questions now being asked of Eugene Stallworth of
Access Graphics by Det. Fred Patterson were becoming much more
pointed. "Isn't it a fact that John Ramsey resented JonBenet's being
in pageants?" was one question that Stallworth, who'd had experience working as a psychologist in the criminal justice field, refused
to answer. The case was heating up nationally, too, thanks in large
part to the CNN interview and to the media's repeatedly showing
footage of JonBenet's pageant performances. Then word went out
that there was a distinct possibility that the victim had also been
sexually assaulted. This added fuel to media fires that were now
brightly burning throughout America.

On Thursday afternoon, January 2, a meeting of a police organization called the Colorado Consortium for Community Policing
took place. Participants were surprised when Boulder chief Tom Koby
attended, though he left early. Denver police chief David Michaud,
who had a detective force of three hundred, followed Koby out of the
room and offered any help his department could provide. Koby
politely thanked him and kept on walking. As the Ramsey case took
on an increasing amount of regional attention, more law enforcement professionals stepped forward to offer assistance.

The next morning, Assistant District Attorney Bill Wise worried
that the media might get a copy of the questions that Linda Arndt
had faxed to Bryan Morgan. Of all the questions, Wise worried
most about Arndt's asking about whether JonBenet had eaten anything later that evening, since a sharp defense lawyer might guess

that the autopsy had revealed something, a something that, indeed, contradicted what the Ramseys had told Arndt on December 26. District Attorney Alex Hunter, on vacation, was briefed by his assistants, Trip DeMuth and John Pickering, on the autopsy report. The lawyers had a different take on the fluid stain found on JonBenet's thigh than Detectives Arndt and Trujillo, who'd concluded that it was semen. The prosecutors wanted to wait for the forensic tests before deciding that John Ramsey was the single prime suspect. Hunter was also advised that Patsy Ramsey had retained her own lawyer, Patrick Burke, who had offices in Boulder and Denver, and that Bryan Morgan's firm had also retained the services of a public relations professional, Pat Korten. This had all been put together very quickly, Hunter thought, and it was becoming obvious that the Ramseys planned to wage a media campaign to win public support for themselves.

John and Patsy Ramsey had returned to Boulder by Saturday, January 4. Pete Hofstram, at the request of the police, had asked Bryan Morgan to help him obtain a second handwriting sample from Patsy Ramsey. The first two samples she had provided, one on the day JonBenet's body was found and another two days later at the justice center, weren't usable since she'd been so sedated when she'd made them. The Ramseys agreed, but only if the sample was provided at a neutral site and not at police headquarters. The couple was anxious to avoid scrutiny by the media, particularly if the images cast them in a defensive posture. Hofstram offered his house in Boulder as a suitable location, and the Ramseys agreed. Once at the house, Patsy was asked to write out the entire text of the ransom note. She did this until she reached the part about her daughter being beheaded and then she broke down and could not continue. John Ramsey objected to his wife's being forced to repeatedly write the same text, and the session ended, with Mr. Ramsey agreeing to provide a third handwriting sample the next day. That evening, Linda Arndt interviewed Sanford and Renee Lucas at their home. Lucas was increasingly troubled by the fact that he had missed finding JonBenet's body when he first searched the Ramseys' basement. He remembered that John Ramsey possibly called out "Oh, my God. Oh, my God," just *prior to* his switching on the small room's light switch, not just afterward. However, this could have been due, Lucas said, to Ramsey's seeing the white blanket, barely visible in the very darkened room.[15] Renee and Sanford Lucas said that Patsy Ramsey seemed a very loving mother to both of her children and that neither Patsy nor John was a heavy drinker, though they each would have a glass or two of wine with a meal. The Lucases agreed to let the police interview their two children, a boy, seven, and a girl, six. Because of the altercation between Lucas and John Ramsey and because he had a key to the Ramsey house, police subsequently took handwriting, hair, blood, fingerprint, and saliva samples from both Sanford and Renee Lucas. Over the course of the next few months, police interviewed this couple a total of eighteen times, many of these at the Lucases' request.

The Ramseys in Boulder were not the only ones finding the media a meddlesome and complicated presence in their lives. The five Boulder detectives still conducting background interviews in the Atlanta area also were hounded by news reporters and photographers. This was a pressure that the Boulder police were not used to, one that was about to cause one of the department's most experienced detectives to be fired from the JonBenet Ramsey investigation. With tempers on edge and the misunderstanding regarding a supposed interview with a journalist, Det. Sgt. Larry Mason, an experienced cop, was regrettably fired. The loss of this veteran dealt a setback to this case.

Over the weekend of January 4–5, police completed their nine-day examination of the Ramsey house. To do this, they had extended their original search warrant three times. The interior of the Ramsey home was enormous, with more than sixty-eight hundred square feet of living space. The huge structure, covered by a red brick, Tudor-style facade, occupied almost all of the half acre it stood upon. The interior of the house reflected Patsy Ramsey's eclectic and extravagant personality, with bright colors in most rooms. The home contained certain tables Patsy claimed to acquaintances had been purchased at Tiffany's in New York, an elite store known for jewelry that does not sell furniture. The Boulder police took out dozens of boxes of evidence and sent much of it to the Colorado Bureau of Investigation and to the FBI laboratory for further analysis. Detectives also took every notepad and pen they found throughout the house. More than eight hundred items were taken into custody, all of them carefully listed. Two of these items were paintings—one from JonBenet's room—pieces of evidence on the backs of which Det. James Byfield had found duct tape, tape strands similar to that found pasted across the dead girl's mouth. Later investigators learned that in 1993 the duct tape was placed on the backs of the paintings by a local photo and frame shop. Police also took three pieces of carpeting from JonBenet's room, a space that also contained two matching English walnut single beds. The room had a porch that overlooked the house's south yard, and there was a small TV set, with its own VCR, and an extensive collection of videos. There were two tall pageant trophies in the room, one standing near a closet jammed with clothes. JonBenet's pageant costumes were found filling the closets in Melinda's bedroom down the hall. Police took all of the sheets, pillowcases, and other bedding items from JonBenet's room. Burke's bedroom was on the same floor, though separated from JonBenet's room by an adjoining playroom. His room contained two TV sets, a VCR, a computer, and a fish tank.

From the house's cluttered basement, police took the suitcase, along with the shards of glass on it, which were found beneath the broken basement window in Burke's train room. Old movie posters adorned that room's walls, and a train set rested on a platform at the room's center. The suitcase under the broken window was not covered with any dust, and it contained only a blanket, one that later was discovered to have semen on it. Subsequent DNA testing established John Andrew Ramsey as the source of this semen. Investigators took the three windows and their framing from the train room, along with the grating above, the same grating where an intact spider's web was discovered on December 26. Moving farther toward the room where JonBenet's body was found, police looked into the storage closet that John Ramsey and Sanford Lucas had examined that afternoon and found a plaque with "Subic Bay" on it, which they took into evidence. Near the room's entrance, police found two partial sets of golf clubs that belonged to John Ramsey. On the door leading into the room, investigators lifted a single palm print, the one that was never identified. Once inside the wine cellar, the detectives discovered a shoe print bearing the logo Hi-Tec in a powdery dust next to where JonBenet's body had been found, and Det. Michael Everett photographed this evidence. Inside the room police found a half dozen partially used cans of interior paint and seven other gallon-size paint cans. Immediately outside the room, investigators had also found several paintings by Patsy Ramsey, a broken wooden paint brush in an artist's paint tray, and other wooden shards nearby. Investigators also took rope and a string from a sled found outside the room. They removed the door to this room and its jamb. Inside the room, police also discovered a safe in the floor, covered with a tarp. Police collected hair and fibers from the room, as well as the pink Barbie nightgown. On a counter further down the hall from this room, police found a red penknife. Before finalizing this exhaustive search, detectives photographed every inch of the house's interior as it looked after so much had been taken away. Late in the month of January, police also obtained a search warrant to look for pornography on any of the computer hard drives they had seized as evidence.

Boulder County District Attorney Alex Hunter arrived from vacation on that Saturday just in time to attend, along with Bill Wise from his office, a meeting with Police Chief Tom Koby and Cdr. John Eller. At the top of the meeting's agenda were the police complaints about the media's criticizing them for the way they'd handled the case. Eller suggested that the district attorney's office had been the source of many leaks. By this time the press knew that JonBenet had suffered a severe head injury and that she had been garroted. They also knew about the $118,000 ransom note demand, the existence of a preliminary practice draft of a ransom note, and that the pad of paper on which both notes had been written came from inside the house. Both the district attorney's office and the police knew that the prosecutors had always been able to deal better with the media than the police. Specifically, all at the meeting were concerned that the media would get their hands on the sixteen questions that Det.

Linda Arndt had sent to John Ramsey's defense lawyer. Bill Wise finally suggested that the press be told that a routine list of "house-keeping" questions had been sent out, queries that were far more innocuous than the ones Arndt had sent. Wise gave "How many times has Federal Express delivered a package [to the Ramsey household]?" as an example, which is what he later told the media. This, the group agreed, was a good strategy, even though it meant misleading the press. Wise cautioned that reporters might already have an idea of what the questions really were. After the meeting, Chief Koby called Hunter and took the district attorney up on a suggestion he had already made, that the district attorney's office use its media expertise to smooth things over between the police and the press.

By this time, almost a full week into 1997, the number of media people in Boulder had swollen well into the hundreds. Many worked for major national magazines, such as *Time* and *Newsweek*. Then there were the television networks with their trucks and equipment, as well as the reporters' recognizable faces. But the police and the district attorney's office weren't the only ones trying to come to grips with the escalating problems presented by the press. That day, Pat Korten, the Ramseys' newly hired public relations man, met with his clients at the Torrells' home. Korten immediately brought up the question of whether John and Patsy Ramsey intended to attend Sunday services at St. John' s Episcopal Church the next day. Patsy Ramsey emphatically said she would, since she wanted to thank all of her friends and fellow worshipers for their support. Korten had hoped he could talk them out of going. He then assured his clients he was setting to work to see that things at church did not get out of control. Before he left the meeting, Korten accepted photos of Jon-Benet in nonpageant settings provided by the Ramseys. He then had to explain to her parents that, since the media already had and was using the pageant photos, it was very unlikely that they would scale down to using everyday photos of JonBenet. The media always wanted to go with the whatever they perceived as most dramatic. After Korten left this meeting, he called the major television networks to suggest ground rules for the next day's services, a call some observers took as an invitation. He then went to visit the Reverend

Rol Hoverstock and suggested that all of his worshipers use a street door leading out of the church, instead of some going out a side door, as was customary. This, Korten said, would simplify matters, and Hoverstock agreed.[16]

The next morning, when the Ramseys arrived at St. John's, there were dozens of photographers and reporters in front of the church. Television satellite vans clogged the adjacent streets. The Ramseys arrived in Frank Torrell's car. Burke had invited a young friend to accompany him to the services. Inside, the Episcopal bishop was there to bless the new members, because the priest who usually performed this ceremony was ill. The bishop told the congregation he also wanted to support the Reverend Hoverstock. After the services were completed, Pat Korten was outside cordoning off the press and public into two columns for the Ramseys to exit through. Before they came out, John and Patsy stood with the bishop, talking to him. Afterward, the family attended the coffee in the parish hall and then left. Members of the congregation were very bitter toward the media, calling them "sharks" and other names. Some later discovered Korten's phone calls and were angry at him, feeling he had manipulated the whole scene.[17] It must not have occurred to them that the press was going to stake out those services that the Ramseys regularly attended, no matter whether the couple showed up or not.

The police began systematically investigating individuals who had emerged as "persons of interest," or, in some cases, as suspects. On Friday, January 3, Boulder detectives Pat Wyton and Nathan Vasquez interviewed Austin O'Rourke, the Santa Claus at the Ramseys' December 23 Christmas party. O'Rourke had become close to JonBenet, John and Patsy had told the police. He had a key to their home, and he'd played Santa at the Ramseys' Christmas parties each year since 1994. During the 1995 party, JonBenet took her chum on a complete tour of the house, one that included the basement and her scrapbooks. She liked to call him "Old Sam." O'Rourke was in frail condition on the night of the 1996 Christmas party, since he'd had open-heart surgery the previous fall. He brought his wife, Ellen,* to the festivities. O'Rourke said he and his wife had stayed at their cabin in the mountains in Nederland, twenty miles west of

Boulder, all of Christmas day and night. On Christmas day, the couple had been visited by their daughter and her husband and, later, by their son and his wife. A number of the O'Rourkes' friends also visited the couple during the day. The husband and wife went to bed about 10:00 PM. Each confirmed the other's account. Police kept O'Rourke on their list of suspects since the couple's alibi was not corroborated by any outside source. Police interest in O'Rourke intensified later on when news reporters discovered that, back in the early seventies, the O'Rourkes' daughter and another teenage girl had been abducted and the other girl had been sexually assaulted. This crime had never been solved, largely because neither girl was able to describe their assailant. Also during the later seventies, Ellen O'Rourke had written a play about a little girl's being murdered in her family's basement. In a subsequent police interview, one that occurred after the couple had returned from Spain and a long-planned vacation, O'Rourke denied telling JonBenet at the family Christmas party that he would visit her late on Christmas night with a special present. Police also pressed Mr. and Mrs. O'Rourke on why they had not volunteered the information about their daughter's abduction and her friend's rape, as well as the topic of Mrs. O'Rourke's play.

As intriguing as they are, these last two facts do not override the fact that O'Rourke was in failing health, and whoever killed Jon-Benet Ramsey must have been strong enough to inflict a powerful blow to her head. O'Rourke, who later went on network television to try to clear his name, died within two years of JonBenet's death. Odd twists of fate, such as JonBenet's reporting that her family's Santa had promised to visit her with a present late on Christmas night, can prove powerful distractions to scientific police work. Let me give you a hypothetical example: Los Angeles is chosen to host the next Summer Olympic Games. During the week prior to the Games, an American airliner explodes over the Pacific Ocean, just off of the coast. The following Saturday, the first night of the Games, a bomb goes off in a busy Olympic Village park, killing one person, wounding many, and terrifying everyone. This, everyone reasons, must be the work of international terrorists. In point of fact, I have just described the series of events that took place in July of 1996, as Atlanta hosted the Summer Games. The bomb was set off by a homegrown right-wing terrorist who was finally captured in the spring of 2003, and TWA Flight 800 exploded because of faulty electrical wiring near its fuel tanks. One last coincidence that ties into the 1996 events: on the Saturday following the July 17 air tragedy, the number 8-0-0 hit the Connecticut Lottery, almost bankrupting that fund. Who can explain things like this? Yet these coincidences do not mean a frail old man was able to sneak his way into the Ramsey house late on Christmas night, to sexually assault the child, to write a bogus ransom note, and to kill her with a powerful blow to the head, and then get away undetected.

Police were also pursuing other major suspects. Burke Ramsey certainly fell into that category. On Wednesday morning, January 8, JonBenet's nine-year-old brother traveled to the Child Advocacy Center in Niwot, where child psychologist Dr. Suzanne Bernhard questioned him. Patsy Ramsey sat sobbing in the next room. Boulder police detectives Linda Arndt, Jane Harmer, and Ron Gosage observed this interview from the next room, behind a one-way window. The two-hour conversation that the three observed proved very inconclusive. During breaks, the police suggested avenues to Dr. Bernhard that she should pursue. Burke did not want to talk about the tragedy, an understandable mind-set. He seemed dazed, even indifferent. The child psychologist gingerly raised the subjects of sexual molestation and other forms of child abuse in the family, and Burke reacted as though there had never been any instances of this. He seemed to be telling the truth, according to both Dr. Bernhard and the detectives. Dr. Bernhard attempted to delve into any secrets that Burke might know, but the boy replied that a fact was no longer a secret if it was told to someone. Police later studied the videotaped interview, carefully arranged with the Ramseys' attorneys, and found no new information in any of it.

Burke Ramsey again became the focus of intense police interest the following spring. After Patsy Ramsey had made her original 911 call before dawn the day after Christmas, she had not completely hung up her phone. For a few tantalizing seconds, police heard background sounds that they could not understand. Detectives sent this tape out to the best electronic experts in the region and, still, save for Patsy Ramsey's sobbing and prayers, nothing more could be made out of the background noise. Then the police discovered a new and expert electronics company, Aerospace Corporation in El Segundo, California, that they provided with a copy of the tape. What came back was worth all of this trouble. When these sounds were brought up many times over, police heard Burke and John Ramsey in an exchange. The child said, "Please, what do I do?" To this, John Ramsey replied, "We're not speaking to you." Finally, Burke is heard to ask, "What did you find?" This discovery was extremely critical. Burke, as Patsy Ramsey had said, was supposed to have slept through the discovery of the ransom note and through the discovery of JonBenet's being missing from her bedroom. Mrs. Ramsey had evidently lied about this, and the boy had also not contradicted that fabrication of the facts. But, why? Did this mean that Burke Ramsey had killed his little sister and his terrified parents had created the ransom note to divert attention away from him? There is one very important footnote to this evidentiary breakthrough. The police got their report back from the West Coast experts in May of 1997. Yet the prosecutor's office was not informed about this bombshell evidence for an entire year.

The legal wrangling over the Ramsey case continued on, as the weeks swept by. The prosecution was able to keep the search warrant and its supporting documents sealed for, first, thirty days or until an arrest, and then another fifteen days. Pete Hofstram's argument was that only the killer or killers knew many of the facts and to open the evidence to public scrutiny would serve only to protect the perpetrators since all of this critical information was public knowledge and not just theirs alone. The media, principally the Denver and Boulder TV outlets, fought these decisions in court, but, for the time being, lost. Meanwhile, the police continued to receive tips from the alarmed general public and to follow up on them. One woman called to report that her on-again, off-again boyfriend, a writer, had been acting suspiciously since the murder. He came home very late Christmas night, she said, his sweater and pants covered with mud.

He became extremely agitated when the couple watched news of the murder the next evening and spent the next day or so pacing about. He had once interviewed an Access Graphics employee for a business story he was doing. Police extensively questioned this individual, who remained a suspect for some time. All of this was a time-consuming process. Since there was no evidence of a forced entry at the Ramsey home and there were no footprints on the lawn outside the home, just what did a muddy sweater and pants have to do with anything connected to the Ramsey case? Unfortunately, the Boulder police followed up on many similar dead-end tips, costing an enormous amount of time and investigative manpower.

At times, some in the media helped to muddy the water. One glaring example: a radio station reported that John Ramsey had confessed to his daughter's murder, a falsehood that had a particularly devastating effect on hundreds of Access Graphics employees. At about the same time in January, Chief Tom Koby held a news conference with only invited local reporters in a room of the Boulder Public Library, which was the headquarters for the city's community access TV channel. Photographers were not allowed into the room and had to use the chief's image on an outer room's TV screen. This infuriated the national media and many of the local reporters who had been working the story. Koby failed to provide any new information and devoted most of his prepared statement on assuring the people of Boulder that they were in no danger. He also denied that John Ramsey had made any kind of a confession. He then defended his department's handling of the case, adding that the Ramsey home was "a large mansion," a reference to their not finding JonBenet's corpse. Koby then criticized the national interest in the case as "sick curiosity in many ways." Koby's standing with the rank and file in his department was not good prior to this news conference, and his appearance that night did not help any. Driven by their union, the police became more and more critical of Koby, still another distraction from the major task before the force: the solving of this murder.

Alex Hunter and Bill Wise met the day after Chief Koby's news conference. Both wanted to avoid the mistakes that the police had been making, and both wanted, if possible, to take the spotlight off of the Boulder police and refocus it on the investigation. The district attorney's office reached out to the Milwaukee police for their guidelines on how they had handled the media during the Jeffery Dahmer case, the serial killer who had cannibalized his victims. Hunter and Wise set to work establishing their own ground rules for the press. The national media had now become a huge and critical problem; especially the tabloids. The *Globe*, one of the biggest of the supermarket tabloids, had received photos of JonBenet Ramsey's autopsy and were preparing to publish them. Dr. Meyer, the coroner, first heard of this when he received a call from an NBC producer who worked for their evening news anchorman, Tom Brokaw. The Boulder police immediately investigated this crime, since providing these photos to the media was a felony. Detectives questioned one man who worked at the camera shop where police had previously processed their photos and where Dr. Meyers's photos were still being developed. This individual failed to pass a polygraph exam and later confessed when the name of a former deputy sheriff who was now a private investigator was mentioned to him. Both he and the former deputy sheriff were prosecuted. The photographer was later convicted of two misdemeanors and the private investigator of a misdemeanor count of obstruction of justice. They were each sentenced to three days in jail, sixty-four hours of community service, and were required to write letters of apology. The detective was also ordered to give the $5,000 he received from the *Globe* to the Boulder district attorney's office, as well as pay a $500 fine. On the subject of ethics, Bill Wise later disclosed the fact that he'd received a number of bribe offers from the tabloids for insider information, offers he turned down with the observation that anyone trying to bribe a public official in Boulder had to be naive.

In their conversations, Hunter and Wise strove to help the police and their own office regain the momentum in this case. Wise, whom I had known and liked for a number of years, called me in mid-January to sound me out on whether I would like to assist on this case. As usual, my calendar was full of other time-consuming commitments, such as a lecture trip to China. And, of course, I was already hard at work on several other major cases as well as teaching responsibilities at the University of New Haven. Bill also mentioned to me that his team was going to reach out to Barry Scheck, my colleague from the O. J. Simpson defense team and a good friend. Up until Wise's call, I did not know anything about the JonBenet Ramsey case beyond what the public had gleaned from the news accounts. Scheck headed the Innocence Project in New York, an organization that has used recently developed DNA evidence to free many wrongly convicted defendants. He is also a professor at the Benjamin N. Cardozo School of Law. The possibility of working with Barry Scheck again intrigued me, and I told Bill Wise to get back to me with Scheck's answer. Alex Hunter and Wise both wondered whether Scheck's presence on the prosecution team would turn off the police, since he had worked so extensively for defendants. Within a few days, Wise called me back to say that Scheck had accepted his offer to assist the prosecution, and I told him that I would do my best to assist. By then I had become very interested in this case. Barry Scheck later told Larry King on CNN that he had declined an offer from the Ramsey family to join their team. Hunter and Wise weren't the only ones adding to their team: at about this time, John and Patsy Ramsey hired ex–FBI agent John Douglas, a renowned profiling expert, adding to their already considerable team of handwriting experts and other investigators.

Coroner John Meyer had more to attend to than excoriating tabloids for offering bribes and recklessly printing autopsy photos. He was preparing his final autopsy report on what caused the death of JonBenet Ramsey. Dr. Meyer noted the fracture of the child's skull, one that had not been visible before he had removed part of the bone. He found subdural hemorrhaging (under the outermost membrane covering the brain) over the right cerebral hemisphere (lobe), along with a film of subarachnoid hemorrhaging (an inner membrane covering the brain) over the entire right cerebral hemisphere (lobe). He also wrote about a lengthy purple bruise, eight inches by one and a half inches, beneath the skull fracture. There was also a bruise at the tip of the right temporal lobe that measured about a quarter inch. The left temporal lobe of the brain had only minimal bruising. Prior to the fatal brain damage, Dr. Meyer had noted that he'd found scattered petechial (the smallest blood vessels) hemorrhages on each lung and on the heart, which suggested death by strangulation. He wrote that there was a red ink, heart-shaped drawing in the palm of JonBenet's left hand. Dr. Meyer opened his report by describing a series of scratches and abrasions on the victim's chin, on the back of her right shoulder, and several other linear hemorrhages across the left shoulder. On the left side of the small of her back, there were two very small, dried abrasions. He also noted the damage to the child's vagina, and he took several swabs from her thighs and her vagina, anus, and mouth. Dr. Meyer locked away the rough draft of his final report in his office safe, aware that a legal battle was brewing over whether or not it should be made public. One other critically important medical report was about to surface: the CBI laboratory's finding that the smear on Jon-Benet's thigh was not semen but blood. This tended to shift the spotlight of suspicion off of John Ramsey, allowing its glare to shine on others in the increasingly small number of individuals who could have committed this murder. The report also indicated that Jon-Benet's body had been wiped clean, leaving behind a faint residue, as well as the increased sense that there had been a sophisticated cover-up.

John Ramsey was known as an individual who appeared unflappable, no matter how serious the business or the personal crisis seemed. Thus, it was particularly interesting to police to receive a call, in mid-January, from the head of security for the McGuckin Hardware store in Boulder. He reported a very upset gentleman named "John" had called his office manager, asking questions about two early-December American Express purchases charged to the card held by Patsy Ramsey. John had said that his bill indicated that, on December 2 and December 9, Patsy Ramsey had made the purchases, the amounts totaling, respectively, $46.31 and $99.88. The caller wanted specifics on what had been purchased. The office manager, of course, recognized the Ramsey name, and she told John that her computer had already dropped those records since they were more than thirty days old. This meant, she told her caller, that he would have to call back since the manager would have to go through those receipts by hand, a time-consuming chore. John agreed to call back in a few days.

The detectives immediately suspected that this was the first John Ramsey had heard about the purchases and that he feared his wife had bought a spool of the thin line used to strangle JonBenet, duct tape, or something else either used in the actual crime or in a cover-up. Police went to McGuckin Hardware the next morning, and the office manager gave them the two receipts, which she'd found the day of the call. Police also placed a tap on the store's phones and awaited John Ramsey's call back, due on January 20. When "John" called back that day, he seemed much more composed. Since Patsy Ramsey had taken out her own American Express card, the number Ramsey provided was not accurate, and he had to fax the store his identification so the office manager could send him the receipts. Unfortunately, the sales slips did not itemize what had been purchased, but did indicate the section of the store where the items purchased were displayed. One of these, the detectives saw, sold rope. Also, the police were not able to trace John Ramsey's call because it was made through a company in Denver that specialized in subverting phone taps, a useful practice when a business was attempting to use the phones to track down a deadbeat former customer. John Ramsey's employing this company only intensified the detectives' suspicions that he knew a great deal more about his daughter's death than he was saying.

Still, there was no plan in place to interview John and Patsy Ramsey, and the legal wrangling continued to intensify. Lawyers for John and Patsy Ramsey were busy attempting to establish guidelines for how the forensic evidence was tested and who from their side would be allowed to observe these tests. Carl Whiteside, head of the CBI, told the prosecutors that he absolutely refused to allow outside observers, a result of his interpretation of Colorado law. This message was conveyed to the defense attorneys, who countered that they wanted John and Patsy Ramsey listed as suspects, to strengthen their chance of being present during the testing. Alex Hunter and the prosecution did not agree to that. At about this time, the CBI's lab also reported that the bloodstains on JonBenet's undergarments contained the DNA of one more person, other than JonBenet, though the majority of the blood came from the victim. The elderly man who lived across the street could not be ruled out as a source, and his boarder was again asked for a handwriting sample, since the first sample he submitted had some resemblance to the ransom note. Boulder police commander John Eller had proposed that the Ramseys be interviewed at 6:00 one evening, with no established end time, an offer the Ramseys' attorneys rejected immediately. Meanwhile, detectives continued to question former Access Graphics employees who had some sort of grievance with the company. In one case, a husband and wife team ended up owing Access Graphics $36,000, which became $18,000 each after they divorced. As noted earlier, this amount was exactly $100,000 less than the ransom note's demand, a fact that intrigued the police. The woman had an airtight alibi for Christmas night, but the man did not. He lingered as a suspect for months, though he did not have a key to the Ramsey house.

Alex Hunter now had to fight off several problems. One was a recommendation by Police Chief Koby to indict John and Patsy Ramsey for their daughter's murder since the police felt that they had enough evidence to establish the probable cause needed for the arrest. Hunter agreed that the probable cause level had been attained, but he argued that the investigation had not come anywhere near a case that was "beyond a reasonable doubt," the level of evidence needed for a conviction. Instead, Hunter told Koby, he wanted the police not just to focus on Mr. and Mrs. Ramsey, but to broaden their investigation. Hunter considered the ransom note the best evidence that the police had. Even here, though, Hunter was worried about the way the courts treat handwriting evidence. He was particularly interested in a hearing in a federal court in Denver on handwriting evidence in the Oklahoma City bombing case against Timothy McVeigh. One of the defense lawyers called handwriting analysis "junk science." Ultimately, District Court Judge Richard Matsch decided to allow expert testimony on the similarities between McVeigh's handwriting and a truck rental contract signed by a fictitious person. However, Judge Matsch also decided that no definitive conclusions by the experts could be allowed into evidence. Police Chief Koby and Cdr. John Eller met with Hunter and top members of the prosecution staff in early February. The police told Hunter, Bill Wise, Pete Hofstram, and the others that they were no longer willing to share information with the prosecutor's office due to the media's receiving so much information via unnamed sources. Thus, the rift between the police department and the Boulder prosecutor's office was now complete, a fact that had a very negative impact on the JonBenet Ramsey murder investigation.

The Boulder police escalated their accusations against Hunter and his staff after any and all news leaks. In mid-February, Hunter met with Chief Koby and advised him that Barry Scheck and I were joining the prosecutor's team. Koby's initial response was negative, a this-is-the-sort-of-thing-we've-been-talking-about response. Then Hunter told Koby that Barry Scheck and I were going to be available to the police, also, and this seemed to make a difference. As a gesture of good faith, Chief Koby agreed to send Det. Tom Trujillo east to my laboratory, with a case report, videotapes, and crime scene photographs, so that I could get started. When he got to Connecticut, Trujillo proved very helpful, and I introduced him to Elaine Pagliaro, my deputy, and other key personnel in our lab. Koby and Hunter also agreed that there should be a common command post where the prosecutor's staff and police could regularly meet. This space, located on neutral ground in the Boulder Justice Center, quickly became known as "the war room." All the case's information was stored in computers with passwords that only the investigators knew. Any information that was exclusively shared by either side was, by agreement, not to leave the room. Finally, Alex Hunter agreed not to involve himself in the day-to-day investigation, working through Pete Hofstram and others, instead. This would, it was hoped, make the police more comfortable and everyone would work together as a team.

Things continued to heat up on the legal front as well as in the media. The news media had retained the services of several First Amendment attorneys in an attempt to have the autopsy report made public. Judge Carol Glowinsky heard arguments in her Justice Center courtroom. Attorneys representing the police and coroner's office argued that the release of the complete autopsy report would cripple an ongoing investigation. In an unusual move, the judge offered to let the plaintiffs' attorneys read the report and affidavits in her chambers, an invitation that was turned down. Finally, Judge Glowinsky, recognizing the public's right to know, agreed to release an amended copy of the autopsy report, one that included the phrase "abrasion and vascular congestion of vaginal mucosa." The coroner's other significant findings from the autopsy on the victim's vagina were excised. Meanwhile, the CBI reported its finding a black pubic hair on the blanket that had covered JonBenet's body when it was found in the wine cellar (the source of which has never been discovered). All the members of the Ramsey family, including John Andrew and Melinda, then agreed to provide samples of their pubic hair. There were many innocent ways that that hair could have transferred to the blanket, such as another person, a family member or not, using the blanket prior to JonBenet's death. It was also possible that the hair was transferred to the blanket while it was being laundered.

The media issue still needed to be addressed. In mid-February, Patsy Ramsey called the Boulder sheriff's office and complained that reporters and photographers were hounding her day and night and she wanted police protection. With her attorney, Patrick Burke, Mrs. Ramsey met with deputies to complain, particularly about an altercation that had led to the arrest of the man at whose house the Ramseys were then staying. This call and meeting, too, made it into the media, though the sheriff's office was quick to say that the "media harassment" issue was the only matter discussed and that Patsy Ramsey had not been asked any questions about the crime itself. Then, on Thursday, February 13, Alex Hunter and Chief Tom Koby held a joint news conference. This time there were literally hundreds of members of the press corps in attendance. Hunter made an opening statement, vowing to find and bring to justice anyone responsible for JonBenet's death. He cautioned the perpetrators of the crime that the circle of suspects was narrowing, that, inexorably, they were going to become the only ones under suspicion, and that they would be brought to justice. Carried live by CNN, Alex Hunter

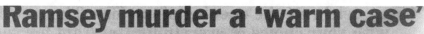

Ramsey murder a 'warm case'

Criminalist discusses
new analysis of forensic
evidence; puzzle appears
no closer to being solved

By Kevin McCullen
News Staff Writer

BOULDER — Famed criminalist Henry Lee called the JonBenet Ramsey murder investigation a "warm case" Thursday.

But, after a half-day meeting with prosecutors, police and analysts Thursday, the 3-year-old murder case appeared no closer to being solved.

Lee, the commissioner of Connecticut's Department of Public Safety, briefed Boulder District Attorney Alex Hunter, special prosecutor Mike Kane and Boulder Police Chief Mark Beckner and his investigators about the latest analysis of forensic evidence in the Dec. 26, 1996, murder.

It was the first meeting between local authorities and Lee since last year. FBI analysts who have reviewed forensic evidence also spoke with the group by telephone.

"We know more now than we did last week," Beckner said.

Beckner, Hunter and Lee — who has advised Hunter on the case since February 1997 —

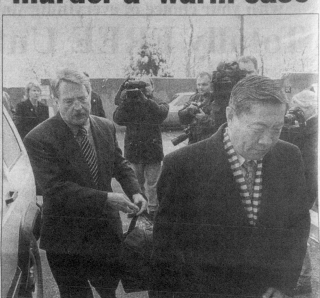

Newspaper article on Dr. Lee's arrival in Boulder to meet District Attorney Alex Hunter to consult on the case.

had quickly become the master face of the investigation. In these opening remarks, Hunter referred to a David-and-Goliath situation, a comment that seemed to intrigue the media, who interpreted Goliath as the wealthy and resourceful Ramsey family. Hunter also took this occasion to announce that Barry Scheck and I had joined his team. Part of the strategy for this news conference was to reestablish a professional relationship with the media.

In his opening remarks, Chief Koby announced that the CBI had completed its DNA analysis and that blood samples were being sent to Cellmark in Maryland, a highly respected laboratory, for further testing. He also endorsed what the prosecutor had said and warned that there was not going to be a quick solution to the case. However, when the reporters began to ask Koby questions, the chief told the mass of reporters that he had been trained not to ever answer any "stupid questions" and that professional reporters knew better than to ask those types of questions in the first place. Koby added that he would not answer any questions that were speculative in nature and, finally, that there would be no information given out that could compromise the investigation. To most observers, Alex Hunter had come off looking like a college football coach and Chief Koby not so well.[18] The following day, Patsy Ramsey called Alex Hunter and thanked him for his fighting words and his commitment to finding her daughter's murderer.

Bill Wise, Hunter's top assistant, had not been present at the news conference since he had to go to a Boulder County commissioners meeting, asking for additional funds for the investigation. The board eventually voted to add $124,000 to the prosecution's budget. There were no members of the press corps covering the meeting. One of the commissioners asked Wise if he had been critical of the Boulder Police Department's work in this investigation. Wise said that he had not yet, but that he was ready to criticize the investigation. He indicated that Alex Hunter's close relationship with Chief Tom Koby was the only reason that the prosecutor's office was at all close to the investigation. Kevin McCullen, a reporter for the *Rocky Mountain News* of Denver, had been at the big news conference, but, as was his reporter's habit, he stopped by the council chambers and listened to Wise's public comments. This soon got back to Wise, who realized that he had spoken out of turn. After consulting with Alex Hunter, Wise called McCullen, who refused to take the comments out of his story. Wise then called his editor, who agreed, for the sake of the investigation, to comply with Wise's extraordinary request. This all backfired, though, when a commissioner told a reporter with the Denver NBC-TV affiliate about the comments and they were broadcast that evening. Bill Wise even attempted to get his quotes back into McCullen's story, but his call to the paper was too late. When Chief Koby heard about what Wise had said, he called Hunter and tried to get Wise removed from the Ramsey case, a request that the prosecutor flatly turned down. In spite of Bill Wise's very public apologies for his remarks, the second objective of the news conference had been shattered: the Boulder Police Department and the county prosecutor's office were again at swordpoint. And the media now increased their coverage of the story, with ABC spending $150,000 a month on it. Both the police and the prosecutor's office were becoming inundated with calls from around the country and even around the world.

With my introduction to the case by Alex Hunter, the media also began to track me down by calling my state police forensic laboratory and my office at the University of New Haven. I was entering the Ramsey investigation more than six weeks after Jon-Benet's body had been discovered. As with the O. J. Simpson case, I knew that I had to obtain any and all information by studying crime scene photos and police reports. On the upside, the CBI and the FBI were now providing their scientific analyses of some of the case's most critical evidence. The fingerprint examiners had been able to identify almost all of the fingerprint evidence that had been recovered by the Boulder police. Unfortunately, no fingerprints were found on the duct tape. There were two prints lifted by the police from the glass bowl that contained the pineapple chunks that were left out on a table in the Ramsey home. One was Patsy Ramsey's, and the other was from her son, Burke. This was perplexing since the coroner had found undigested pineapple chunks in the victim's upper colon. Considering the family's statement that they returned home on Christmas night around 10:00 and that Jon-Benet was already asleep and was directly carried upstairs and put to bed by John Ramsey, this meant that either JonBenet's mother or her brother had probably given her the pineapple as a snack, either before she went to bed or later that night before her death. And, of course, this underscored that, for some reason, the family had, in all likelihood, not been truthful about their daughter's being asleep and put directly to bed. The fingerprint examiners were unable to identify the palm print left on the door to the basement wine cellar where JonBenet's body was discovered.

As noted before, the CBI had also determined that the stain on JonBenet's underpants was blood and that it contained DNA from another source. The CBI used a PCR (Polymerase Chain Reaction) marker to establish this fact, though the blood samples had been sent on to Cellmark in Maryland for the more precise RFLP

(Restricted Fragment Length Polymorphism) testing that would take at least another month to complete. Armed with this new information, police detectives questioned JonBenet's playmates on whether any ever exchanged clothes with her, and one said that she and Jon-Bonet had worn each other's clothing. Also, they discovered that Sanford Lucas had sometimes changed JonBenet when she had soiled herself. The FBI laboratory had reported that they were working on identifying the manufacturer of the duct tape found covering JonBenet's mouth and might even be able to find when the tape was manufactured and where it had been purchased. The FBI had also found four fibers on the tape, red and black, and they were attempting to identify the source of these fibers. Thus, from a scientific standpoint, I was entering the case just as things were heating up. Coincidentally, the FBI expert who was working so diligently on this investigation was Douglas Deedrick, the special agent who had testified in the O. J. Simpson case, an expert I had worked with on several earlier cases.

Alex Hunter continued to steer the Ramsey investigation toward the center of the road, resisting calls for a grand jury investigation. In one news conference, he called himself "Mr. Evidence," an obvious reference to the increasing outcry for an arrest in this case. With so much of the forensic evidence still out being tested, this was a wise strategy. The relationship between the Boulder police and the prosecutor's office continued to deteriorate, and "the war room" established as a mutual workplace fell into disuse. Meanwhile, as the winter of 1997 turned into spring, the media continued to hound any or all individuals who were in any way associated with the investigation. Each time a new fact surfaced, such as the CBI's establishing that the same pad as the one found in the Ramsey home used for the ransom note was also used for a practice note, the press and public interest seemed to erupt anew. Once the entire note itself finally became public, everyone under the sun seemed to have an opinion or insight to offer. For instance, it was accurately reported that several of the phrases used, such as "I don't care if it's a Pekinese pissing against a lamppost," were from *Dirty Harry*, a seventies movie that starred Clint Eastwood. Also, in the movie *Speed*, Dennis

Hopper warns the authorities, "Do not attempt to grow a brain." At 7:30 on the night of December 25, a Boulder channel broadcast the movie *Nick of Time*, in which a political terrorist group kidnaps a six-year-old girl, using the phrase "Listen to me carefully." The actual handwriting analyses by the CBI and other expert consultants were inconclusive, though most ruled out John Ramsey as the note's author, but there were indications that the handwriting was similar to that of Patsy Ramsey. Later on, an individual stepped forward who purported to be an expert on analyzing writers' voices, and he claimed that the voice of the ransom note was that of Patsy Ramsey. If handwriting analysis is difficult and indistinct, how much more nebulous is the establishment of a writer's voice in a specific piece of writing?

Meanwhile, the Boulder police continued to follow up on many leads. One was the entire pageant world. Detectives fanned out and questioned dozens of individuals who had either directly dealt with the Ramsey family or knew this area well. Nothing important was found. Then there was the question of whether JonBenet had been sexually abused prior to her death. Police questioned area prostitutes on whether John Ramsey had ever been a customer or otherwise active in the world of pornography. The answer, again, was a resounding no. The FBI concluded that the sexual trauma to JonBenet Ramsey seemed intended to mislead investigators. Whether before or after her death, the sexual assault was not consistent with anything that would have provided gratification to the perpetrator. Like Alex Hunter, the FBI profilers felt that the ransom note was the case's most important piece of evidence and that, whenever it was written, the note itself represented the case's most time-consuming action by the perpetrator. Investigators found that even the way the rope was applied to the victim's neck was very unusual. Since the rope and the abrasion ran around her neck in an even fashion, there was no real evidence of any kind of a struggle. This kind of weapon to kill a child was unprecedented. Most telling, they concluded, by leaving the body in a location where it would be quickly discovered, the perpetrators contradicted the ransom note since this discovery eliminated any possibility of a financial payoff.

By late winter, the facts and forensic evidence had been extensively investigated and the findings had become established. Working with Alex Hunter, I had to review thoroughly all of these findings and then provide him with the best analysis possible. Meanwhile, the feud between the prosecutor's staff and the police intensified. The Boulder police actually hired their own attorney to advise them in their investigation. Also, Police Chief Tom Koby was subject to increased criticism by the rank-and-file police and the detectives who were working the Ramsey case. The police gave their chief a vote of no confidence during the spring and followed up with a second similar vote in the summer. Koby was under constant fire, and the feeling developed that he could not survive much longer in his position. The Boulder chief did not help his cause when, after a large student riot in early May at the University of Colorado, Koby declared that his men would have been justified in killing some of the rioters in self-defense.[19] Rather than help his relationship with his force, these remarks angered many in the media and the general public. Many times, police and fire department officers develop resentment for their chiefs, who are, essentially, their bosses. Their unions often help to spur on this activity. The sad fact is that this dissension in the Boulder police ranks served to work against the solution of the JonBenet Ramsey murder. Of course, the continued presence of hundreds of national and local journalists did not help the situation, either. It is hard for public officials to do their jobs when they are looking over their shoulders constantly or, worse, preoccupied with talking to reporters who promise them anonymity for their insights.

Negotiations between Alex Hunter's office and the Ramseys' lawyers continued. The attorneys insisted that John and Patsy Ramsey be provided with transcripts of their earlier statements to investigators and that the interrogations take place in the couple's lawyers' offices. Hunter felt this was reasonable, but these concessions, when made, infuriated the police, who also resented the fact that Pete Hofstram of the district attorney's office had met four times over breakfast with John Ramsey's attorney, Bryan Morgan. It was well into the spring, and the police still had been unable to individually sit down across from JonBenet's parents, now considered

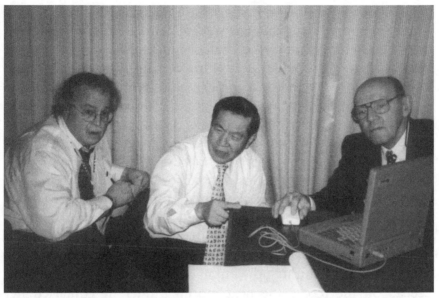

Dr. Michael Baden (left), Investigator Lou Smit (right), and Dr. Lee (center) examine and review evidence.

prime suspects, to interrogate them. The two sides set April 23 as a date for the negotiated interviews. Lou Smit was a retired Colorado Springs detective whom Alex Hunter hired to assist in the investigation. Studying the autopsy photos, Smit noted two sets of aligned abrasions, one on the victim's lower back and a second just below her right ear, set close together, that looked as though they had been left there by a stun gun. There had been a 1993 child homicide case in Colorado in which police had convicted a mother and her boyfriend of murdering her little girl, a crime that had included the use of a stun gun. When Smit consulted the Boulder coroner, Dr. John Meyer said that he could not say for certain that the marks came from such a weapon, but allowed that this was possible. Other experts agreed. The investigators hired by the Ramseys argued that JonBenet's parents could not possibly have resorted to the use of a stun gun in the commission of her homicide. Like so much other evidence in this case, the entire debate led to an inconclusive outcome.

Because he was being deluged by calls from the media, Alex Hunter also hired a special press representative. He would need this help. Just prior to the April 23 interviews scheduled for John and Patsy Ramsey, the Boulder police, led by Cdr. John Eller, aborted those meetings. On April 22, the FBI's Child Abduction and Serial Killer Unit had advised the Boulder police that, under the negotiated circumstances, it was highly unlikely that any productive results could be derived from those sessions. This all led to an angry letter from the Ramseys' attorneys to Alex Hunter, which, when publicized, led to a public relations disaster for both the police and the prosecutor's office. Headlines and broadcasters sensationalized this latest twist in the investigation. Patsy Ramsey called Phil LeBeau, a reporter with a large Denver TV channel, the afternoon of the twenty-third and agreed to tell him that this action was what the couple had been putting up with all along. She agreed to speak to LeBeau on the record the next morning, after he contacted her through a third party. The next evening, LeBeau went on the air with his exclusive story. Mrs. Ramsey said, "We'll sit and talk with them [the police] twenty-four hours, if that's what they want. . . . You'd think if they think we're guilty, they'd want to talk to us." John Eller then took to the media to spell out what his investigators required for a realistic and productive interview. On April 25, the *Denver Post* published a list of police demands, which included the following: separate, taped interviews for Mr. and Mrs. Ramsey, starting with Patsy Ramsey; an open-ended time limit would be established; and the interviews would be conducted by two Boulder detectives, selected in consultation with Alex Hunter. "Standard police interview techniques" would be used, and the interviews would be held at a suitable neutral site, such as the Child Advocacy Center in Niwot, where Burke had been interviewed. Negotiations were restarted and, finally, April 30 was set as the new date for the long-awaited police interviews of John and Patsy Ramsey. Over the weekend prior to the new Ramsey interview date, the couple ran an ad in the Boulder paper, the *Daily Camera*, offering a reward of $100,000 for anyone providing information that directly led to the arrest and conviction of JonBenet Ramsey's killer.

Attorneys for John and Patsy Ramsey arrived at Mr. Ramsey's Access Graphics office the afternoon before the scheduled questioning, where John Ramsey awaited them. Patsy Ramsey arrived a short while later, though she did not remain in the office throughout the lengthy strategy session that lasted until 6:00 PM. At the Boulder police headquarters, detectives met with members of the FBI's Child Abduction and Serial Killer Unit for advice on how to proceed. Then Dets. Steve Thomas and Ron Gosage met with Pete Hofstram to discuss strategy. Par for the course, Hofstram cautioned against the questioning being too rough, particularly at the outset, saying that he wanted to see the Ramseys won over. Thomas and Gosage disagreed. The two detectives wanted to lock JonBenet's parents into a story so that, as events unfolded, the couple would be trapped into a single account of events. The police intended to catch Mrs. Ramsey in contradictions similar to her contrasting accounts on when she had first checked her daughter's room the morning of December 26. Patsy Ramsey initially said that she'd found JonBenet missing from her bed before she went downstairs. Later, she'd told Det. Linda Arndt that she'd gone straight downstairs, without checking on Jon-Benet before she found the ransom note. To accomplish their objective, Thomas and Gosage had decided to avoid asking about the pineapple chunks in the victim's upper intestine and to withhold other critical information, such as the taped evidence from the 911 call. The police were preparing to play hardball.

The next morning, shortly after 9:00, Patsy Ramsey sat in the district attorney's conference room at the Boulder Justice Center, across from Dets. Steve Thomas and Tom Trujillo. Her attorney, Pat Furman, sat in a chair next to his client. An investigator for the Ramsey family also was in the room, as was Pete Hofstram. This questioning went on for six hours, with only a short lunch time-out and a couple of bathroom breaks. Patsy Ramsey told them that her daughter had been asleep when they arrived home from the Lucas house and that she was put directly into bed. The little girl had not awakened. Then she was asked about the last thing that JonBenet had eaten that night, a question she had already answered in writing in response to Linda Arndt's submitted queries. Now, she said she didn't remember, though earlier she had written "cracked crab" from the Lucas home in her answer to Arndt's question. Later on, after a short break, Trujillo returned to this question, and Mrs. Ramsey then remembered about the cracked crab meal at the Lucas home. She was next specifically asked if any family member had eaten anything on their return home, and Mrs. Ramsey said she did not remember anyone doing so. Mrs. Ramsey must have known about the pineapple from the autopsy report during this interview, since that information had been released in the edited version of the autopsy. Mrs. Ramsey also insisted, under repeated questioning, that Burke had slept through the early morning events and awoke only when his father got him up to go over to the Lucas house.

The detectives pressed Mrs. Ramsey on the ransom note, asking why some experts felt that the writing resembled hers. She said that could be the case if a woman wrote the note. When they asked how she could explain the note's being written by a felt-tipped pen she owned, she said that that was the first she'd heard about this fact and she did not have an opinion. The detectives questioned Mrs. Ramsey on what she wore on the morning she discovered her daughter was missing from her room, and she described the red sweater and black slacks she'd worn to the Lucas party the night before, since these clothes were handy when she woke up. This questioning pertained to the black fibers found on the duct tape, JonBenet's body, the white blanket, and the floor of the wine cellar. The detectives were also aware that Mrs. Ramsey was known for her meticulous attention to her appearance, being a person who did not leave her bedroom each morning without her makeup applied. Wearing the same clothing two days in a row seemed out of character for her. When she was asked if she would take a polygraph test, Mrs. Ramsey said, "I'll take ten of them." In subsequent days, Mrs. Ramsey's lawyers and Pete Hofstram were not able to agree on ground rules for the polygraph test, and none was ever administered. During the breaks, Mrs. Ramsey, with Pete Hofstram's consent, was allowed to talk privately with her lawyers, a practice that bothered the detectives, since they were afraid the lawyers would be passing her answers on to John Ramsey. Patsy Ramsey said that she did not remember buying a roll of duct tape, either locally or in Georgia. This critical interview ended in midafternoon. The detectives had found Mrs. Ramsey calm and very much in control of herself and her answers, even a little bit charming.

John Ramsey followed his wife into the conference room to answer questions from Detectives Thomas and Trujillo. Bryan Morgan, his attorney, sat in a chair next to him. Just as they had with Patsy Ramsey, the detectives carefully walked Ramsey through the previous statements he had made. He was asked about the discrepancy between his saying he had taken a sleeping JonBenet directly up to her bedroom and his telling Rick French, the first officer on the scene, that he had read to her before she had fallen asleep. Ramsey replied that he'd meant to say he had retired to read, himself. With their exclusive knowledge of Burke Ramsey's voice on the background of the 911 call, the detectives listened as Ramsey reiterated his statement that his son had slept through the traumatic predawn events of that morning and that he'd awoken Burke at 7:00 to take him to the Lucas residence. John Ramsey did, however, provide new information on that morning to the detectives when he surprised them by saying he'd made his own private trip into the basement at 10:00 AM. He then told the police that he had found the broken window in the train room open. Steve Thomas asked Ramsey why he had not reported the open window, since this could have been an access point for the assailants. John Ramsey replied that he simply didn't know why he'd kept quiet about what he'd found. He also said that his basement visit did not extend to the boiler room or the wine cellar.

The detectives had already conducted tests on the ambient and reflected light in the wine cellar where the victim's body was found. These tests, made by the owner of a local camera shop, indicated that there was not enough light in the room for an average person at the door to see the white blanket and JonBenet's hands protruding out from under it. However, they'd found, since the body was to the left of the entrance, if a person stood five to ten inches inside the room, more light would have been in evidence, enough, perhaps, for Ramsey to see the blanket and body. This could have been the reason why Sanford Lucas had not seen the body when he made his search that morning and why John Ramsey, before he'd turned on the room's light switch, had been able to see the blanket and hands. Trujillo and Thomas wanted to know why Ramsey had called his private pilot just twenty minutes after discovering the body and had started arranging an immediate flight to Atlanta. Ramsey said that he felt his family was in danger in Boulder and that Atlanta would be safer for them. Ramsey became very angry with the detectives when they asked him if he would take a lie detector test. "I have never been so insulted in my life as by that question," he said. Thomas then bluntly asked if Ramsey would take one. "No," came the answer. The detectives wrapped up their interview with John Ramsey after only two hours, one-third of the time they devoted to questioning his wife. Neither interview had provided much concrete, new information. Alex Hunter was briefed on the interviews the next day.

Reporters had been tipped off about the Ramseys facing their first real interviews with the police. Most who staked out the Justice Center building that day were disappointed. Some caught a glimpse of John Ramsey slipping into the building around 3:00 PM. The Boulder police put out a statement saying that it "had been a full day." But the Ramsey family was not now going to slip back into silence. Their press representatives began calling a select few Boulder and Denver reporters about a news conference that the couple was going to hold the next afternoon, Thursday, May 1, though the session's whereabouts remained cloaked in secrecy. The seven reporters were each given a password and instructions on where to go and whom to meet. All seven eventually found themselves in a suite at the Marriott Hotel in Boulder, where the press reps gave them more ground rules. There would be no questions directed at either John or Patsy Ramsey on whether either of them had murdered their daughter, and the session would not last longer than a half hour. The Ramseys' lawyers were going to be present, and, while TV cameras were allowed, no still photographs could be taken. Then John and Patsy Ramsey came into the room and started the discussion by explaining why they had each retained counsel. John Ramsey said that the couple had been anxious to meet the media for some time, but that they did not feel comfortable doing that before each had sat down and had given the police complete interviews. Mr. Ramsey volunteered that he did not kill his daughter and added that the innuendoes about her being sexually molested were false and that these were "the most hurtful innuendoes to us as a family." He concluded this by saying, "I will miss her dearly for the rest of my life."

Patsy Ramsey, looking poised, sat next to her husband as he carried the first portion of the discussion. Mrs. Ramsey, when her husband had completed his remarks, expressed her gratification that she was talking to the media, face to face, and said, "I'm appalled that anyone would think that John or I would be involved in such a hideous, heinous crime." She then also denied that she had killed her little girl. John Ramsey then added that he'd been receiving a great deal of support in the mail from the American general public, one set of letters from a lady, eighty-five, who had to wait for her Social Security check before buying postage for her letter. "It's just been wonderful," he concluded. Patsy Ramsey then said that the couple "appreciated some of what you've said. I'll be frank, not all of what you've said." She then implored the media, "We need to work together as a team," and she cited the recently advertised $100,000 reward. To end her prepared statement, Mrs. Ramsey said that she thought there were at least two individuals who knew who killed her daughter, the killer and someone he or she had "confided in." She hoped that "just one phone call" would come in to solve the crime. In answer to a reporter's question, John Ramsey said that the couple had been communicative with the police, saying the impression that the couple had resisted talking to the police was "totally false," and cited their statements of December 26 and 27. He said he was insulted when his wife and he had become suspects and that any further police questioning was "a waste of time," since they had not committed the crime. John Ramsey was asked if there was anything he wanted to say to JonBenet's killer. "We'll find you. We will find you. I have that as a sole mission for the rest of my life." Patsy Ramsey endorsed her husband's comments: "You may be eluding the authorities for a time, but God knows who you are and we will find you." Mrs. Ramsey addressed her remarks directly at the television cameras and poked her finger to provide emphasis. Both

Mr. and Mrs. Ramsey, when asked, endorsed the death penalty as punishment for their daughter's killer, when convicted. Their press aide abruptly ended the news conference a short time later.

The Ramseys at this point had very effectively taken the offensive. The couple came out of the police interviews unscathed and then followed up with this news session, which many in the media quickly dubbed a Ramsey family infomercial. Given some obvious jealousy from the hundreds of reporters who were not asked to attend, this judgment does not seem that harsh. Media analysts particularly discussed Patsy Ramsey's habit of shutting her eyes when she spoke, something that made it appear to them that she was lying.[20] Then there is the timing of these two events to consider. After getting through the long-awaited police interviews, the Ramseys' timing for their addressing the media seemed right on. John and Patsy Ramsey were also taking other steps to go on with their lives. The couple began planning to sell their home in Boulder and to return to the Atlanta area, where they would have relatively less exposure to the media and to others seeking to intrude into their daily lives. Their son, Burke, had a much better chance for a normal childhood away from Boulder. Also, John Ramsey did not seem able to throw himself back into his duties as chief executive at Access Graphics and he had begun to signal to Lockheed Martin, the parent company, that he wanted to move on. Lockheed Martin, in turn, began to reevaluate its ownership of Access Graphics, and later sold its subsidiary.

John and Patsy Ramsey also likely began to sense that Alex Hunter and the district attorney's office were attempting to broaden the investigation in solving their daughter's murder, more than the Boulder police. Lou Smit, the investigator hired by Hunter, was particularly outspoken about his wanting to follow the trail of evidence, no matter where it led, and this, combined with his outspoken Christian beliefs, seemed to encourage the Ramseys. The couple also continued to press their advertising campaign. An ad published in mid-May also tied them to the district attorney's office. Appearing on Sunday, May 11, in the Boulder paper, the *Daily Camera*, the ad again offered $100,000 as a reward and specifically called for apprehending "an adult male approaching young children in late 1996."

Reporters got wind of this ad prior to its publication, and their digging revealed the fact that this alleged suspect was well dressed and Caucasian. When asked, Hunter's press representative initially denied any cooperation by the district attorney's office in preparing the advertisement. This disclaimer proved wrong, as Hunter found out from defense lawyer Bryan Morgan the day before the ad's publication, during a chance encounter at a children's soccer game. In actuality, Hunter's deputy, Trip DeMuth, had been shown the copy for the advertisement and had given the copy his approval. This fact, when it became known, only served to deepen the impression that the district attorney's office was fully cooperating with John and Patsy Ramsey, a feeling that was reinforced when the Ramseys publicly thanked Hunter and his staff for their help.

Meanwhile, problems for the Boulder police seemed to be compounding. On May 10, a man was shot to death by an ex-girlfriend as a police officer stood outside by the door. The victim had called ahead and asked for police protection as he removed his belongings from his former residence. Things seemed to be going smoothly enough until the fatal gunfire. This incident proved very embarrassing. The police also formally took Det. Linda Arndt off the case, along with another female detective. The Colorado media had become increasingly critical of the Boulder police force's work on the Ramsey case, and much of the criticism focused on Arndt. There was a false report that the detective had been the one to move the little girl's dead body from the basement to the living room and that she had, without permission, given a copy of the ransom note to a defense lawyer. When Arndt asked Cdr. John Eller to back her up on this and other falsehoods, Eller refused. To her credit, Detective Arndt remained silent throughout these media attacks on her.[21]

In late May, Alex Hunter won a four-month extension on the court-ordered seal protecting the contents of the original search warrants for the Ramsey residence. Judge Diane MacDonald, noting the harm that the release of certain information could bring to the investigation, said that "there can be no more compelling governmental interest than the arrest and prosecution of her [JonBenet Ramsey's] killer." Hunter, at the suggestion of his press aide, was also beginning to take the offensive in his attempts to put the Ramsey investigation in the best light. The media, meanwhile, continued to press for the release of the complete autopsy report, a case that the county attorney's office was defending. A lower court ruled in favor of the full report's release, but the county appealed this ruling to the Colorado Supreme Court, and this, effectively, meant that portions of the autopsy would remain sealed until a final ruling. In the meantime, the police continued to pursue their leads. Investigators found an employee at the Denver-based telephone security firm that had made the calls to the McGuckin Hardware store who said that the original caller was a fellow employee who had impersonated John Ramsey. This same individual had also, in January, lifted Ramsey's signature from his bank records and had subsequently faxed this to the store. While none of this was ever prosecuted, for fear of having the case's records ordered opened, the investigators found that the original customer for the Denver company was a tabloid TV reporter. The police, at this point, were faced with a labyrinth of material to investigate, much of it media-driven and only a small percentage of it valuable to the case.

I again went out to Boulder in late May to meet with Alex Hunter and his key people, along with Detectives Thomas, Trujillo, Harmer, and Gosage, who were central to the Ramsey investigation. We combed over a list of the items in the Ramsey house that needed specific attention, if and when there would be another search there. This meeting was also designed to provide an open and candid exchange of opinions on the case and to provide any new information. During this conference, I emphasized the importance of determining the following issues:

- the source and amount of pineapple in JonBenet's system and its degree of digestion, and whether or not the time when she ate the pineapple could be established
- the time of the blow to JonBenet's head in relation to the timing of the ligature application and her vaginal injury
- the source of the duct tape, the ligature, and the traces of wood fragment found in her vagina

- the time of her being garroted and the ultimate time of her death
- the source of the fingerprints found on a teacup and the bowl on the table
- the source of the Hi-Tec boot print found on the floor of the wine cellar

These, I knew, were very difficult facts to establish, and I recommended several excellent forensic pathologists for the police and/or the prosecution to consult. The police, at this time, were receiving a steady stream of forensic test results from the CBI, though not all of this information was being shared with the district attorney's office and me. Except for inconsequential physical samples in the house from John and Patsy Ramsey, these results did not contain any positive identifying information. The handwriting experts at the CBI reported that there were similarities in Patsy Ramsey's writing samples to the ransom note and that she could not be ruled out as the note's author. However, other handwriting consultants could not identify Patsy as the author of the note. The note was not enough, Alex Hunter knew, for an arrest. Even with a positive identification, this only went toward proof of Patsy Ramsey as an accessory after the fact to the crime, and, under Colorado laws, an accessory could not be arrested unless the principal to the crime had already been charged. As I left Boulder, I sensed that the case had hit an impasse, and I heard more and more talk about a grand jury being convened to bring the investigation to a conclusion, a move that Alex Hunter was considering.

As the investigation continued, most of the leads police were pursuing did not provide any payoff for the investigators. Accounts of what was happening often reached Hunter and his office through the media. Reporters had stumbled onto the fact that police were pursuing a link between the ransom note and Psalm 118 from the Old Testament. The oddball $118,000 figure demanded for JonBenet's safe return was one obvious tie-in. However, police had also found John Ramsey's Bible opened on a desk in his home office, turned to Psalm 118. Verse 27 within that Psalm was even more intriguing. In part, it declares, "God is the source, which hath shewed us the light: Bind the sacrifice with cords, even unto the horns of the altar." This seemed a compelling reference to the cord tied around the victim's neck and wrist and the posed manner in which she had been left. Also, a tabloid newspaper revealed that a few years earlier Patsy Ramsey had studied a book, *Healed of Cancer*, by the writer Dodie Osteen. In the text, Osteen refers to Psalm 118, not to verse 27, but to verse 17, which says, "I shall not die, but live, and declare the works of the Lord." Also, a year or so earlier, Patsy Ramsey had talked about her reliance on this book in an interview in *Colorado Woman News*.

Investigators continued to pursue the possibility that JonBenet Ramsey had been the victim of a stun gun applied in two different places on her body. As mentioned earlier, Dr. John Meyer, the coroner, had declared that the marks could not be ruled out as those left by a stun gun. Dr. Robert Deters, a pathologist who had worked a 1988 murder involving a stun gun, was consulted. Did the use of such a weapon paralyze a child of six? Yes, said Dr. Deters. The victim would not even be able to scream. Det. Jane Harmer, with a prompt from the district attorney's office, reinterviewed Brian Scott, the Ramsey family gardener who had become a chum of JonBenet's. Besides rechecking his alibi, Harmer asked Scott about a ridge of grass that had grown below the grating over the train-room window, the one that John Ramsey said he had broken months earlier to get back into the house when he'd found himself locked out. Studying photos, Scott said that the grass had probably grown back under the grate when it had been moved upward, though he could not tell if that was two months earlier or only since the time of JonBenet's death. Scott's girlfriend later told Harmer that he'd returned home around 12:30 on the morning of December 26, so he was not cleared until after his hair, saliva, and handwriting samples had been analyzed.

In late June, I was a guest on CNN's *Larry King Live* show. Larry King is not only extremely intelligent but he's also a very sharp interrogator. When Larry pressed me about the status of the Ramsey investigation, I replied that solving a case was like building a table, one that needed four strong legs. Those legs are a strong investigative team, good forensic evidence, witnesses, and a little bit of luck. Then Larry asked me how many legs of the table we had. I replied: "So far, I would say, they have only one and a half. Maybe."

With the Ramseys planning to move back to Atlanta, the couple signed a consent order in mid-June permitting the police unlimited access to their home. After Burke was finished with school, the family retired to their home in Michigan to spend the summer. The Ramseys asked the investigator Lou Smit, whom they sensed was a kindred spirit, to keep an eye on their property while they still owned it, which Smit did. Later in the summer, John Ramsey wrote to Smit and informed him of his having committed adultery when he was married to his first wife, "the worst thing" he had ever done.[22] Ramsey wanted Smit to know this before he read about it in a tabloid newspaper. Smit then made it a practice to drive by the Ramsey house at seven each morning, where he said a silent prayer for JonBenet. Lou Smit worked closely with the Boulder police detectives, particularly Steve Thomas, in the coming weeks.

On June 30, the investigators combed through the fifteen-room structure. In the evening, some stood outside watching, while others turned the inside and outside lights on and off. One detective stood in a remote corner of the basement and screamed as loudly as possible, while another investigator stood in the opposite end of the house to measure what could be heard loudly enough to awaken a sleeping family. Detectives climbed up and down the thirteen steps of the spiral staircase leading downward from the landing outside JonBenet's bedroom door to the kitchen door. This was especially tricky for them when the stairwell was darkened. The detectives found it was impossible to climb over the bottom steps above the kitchen in a normal fashion without stepping on the spots where the ransom note had been left. The only way to avoid the areas where the three pages had been left was to cling to one wall and to move down in an acrobatic fashion. Yet Patsy Ramsey had not stepped on the note's pages and had not said anything about making any extraordinary moves to avoid the white, lined pages, which did not show any footprints on them. The detectives also attempted to reenact the possible routes through which an assailant could have chased a terrified and screaming little girl. The wine cellar where the body was found was down a corridor, past a utility sink and the boiler room. If JonBenet were running there in fear of her life, an intruder would have had to be in very close pursuit to be able to find the wine cellar in a darkened basement. The investigators combed the house for weeks, yet they never found a roll of duct tape or any kind of object that could have inflicted the fatal skull fracture, except for the flashlight that had sat, without any fingerprints, on a kitchen counter. Someone would have had to either have fled the crime scene with this weapon and tape or left the house in the dead of night and disposed of them.

In July the Ramseys moved their remaining possessions out of their house in Boulder and moved into a residence in an Atlanta suburb, not far from the cemetery where JonBenet was buried. The investigation into the little girl's death had again seemed to have ground to a standstill. Nothing new came out of the exhaustive police investigation at the house, which the family put up for sale at $1 million. On July 12, John and Patsy Ramsey returned to the Boulder Justice Center and met there with Lou Smit and Pete Hofstram. A defense lawyer was also present for the tape-recorded interview. Smit questioned the Ramseys about their ever owning a stun gun, and only John Ramsey vaguely mentioned that once, in Florida, he had been lectured on this weapon and its use for self-defense. The couple also did not own any Hi-Tec shoes, they said, a follow-up question by Smit on the shoeprint found in the dusty floor of the wine cellar, near JonBenet's body. A few days later, Smit asked the same questions of John Andrew Ramsey, with the same results. The stun gun question had, by now, blossomed into another controversy between Lou Smit and the Boulder police detectives. There was even talk of exhuming JonBenet's remains, but Alex Hunter opposed this step because he did not have a great deal of faith in the marks being from a stun gun and he knew the media storm that such a move would cause. Smit openly questioned whether JonBenet's parents could ever use such a device on their six-year-old. This opinion gets past the possibility that someone attempting to stage a sexual crime may have mutilated the victim's sexual organs, post mortem, an equally grisly step. The Boulder police were quick to note that no one from their department was present at either interview.

This lack of investigative progress did not dampen the public's interest in this case, a fascination that was reflected by the enormous amount of media attention. On July 14 the attention to the case intensified more when the Colorado Supreme Court decided that the full autopsy report would immediately be made public. Questions rapidly emerged about the severity of the blow to the victim's head as well as the evidence of damage to her hymen and the traces of blood found in her vagina. A nationally recognized expert on sexual abuse to children, Dr. Richard Krugman, dean of the University of Colorado Health Science Center, had been consulting with the Boulder police and district attorney's office since March. He was quickly placed at the center of this firestorm of interest. Dr. Krugman said that, from what he'd read in the autopsy, JonBenet had not been sexually abused. He explained this finding by adding that physical evidence alone cannot determine whether a child has been the victim of sexual abuse. Along with the child's testimony, such a determination could be established when physical evidence was found, such as semen or a sexually transmitted disease. Krugman also distinguished between physical abuse, such as corporal punishment connected to toilet training, and sexual abuse, which was the result of another's sexual gratification. Then there was the child's medical history to be considered. Krugman's analysis set off another wave of controversy. Dr. Cyril Wecht, an old and respected friend of mine, flatly refuted Dr. Krugman, saying on network television that, with the physical evidence, it was impossible to conclude that JonBenet Ramsey had not been sexually assaulted. Others agreed. John and Patsy Ramsey, through their attorneys, released a statement holding that Dr. Krugman's findings bore out what they had been saying all along, that their daughter had not been sexually assaulted prior to the night of her death. The release of the full autopsy report stimulated the media to appeal Judge Diane MacDonald's finding that the search warrants were to remain sealed. Within a few days, a court upheld Judge MacDonald's decision, and the warrants were kept from public view.

Alex Hunter was disappointed that the Boulder police were not following through on many of the suggestions that I had made to them. Then John and Patsy Ramsey stepped up their advertising campaign. In an open letter published in area newspapers, the couple, based on their own profiling expert's findings, described the suspect as someone the family knew and an individual who had difficulty dealing with females. Also, he was someone who would have acted in a peculiar fashion before and after the crime and who had created some sort of alibi. The FBI and other profilers criticized this description since they contended that there was absolutely no link with it and any of the physical evidence. Meanwhile, the Boulder police decided to ask the FBI for their help and sent files and some of the evidence to the bureau's facilities in Quantico, Virginia, where there would be a conference in early September. Alex Hunter planned to go and to bring along Pete Hofstram, his lead prosecutor, to this conference. Some in the media hailed this joint effort as evidence that the district attorney's office and the police were learning to work together. However, word began circulating in the media that the police, led by John Eller, were planning to take the highly unusual step of retaining their own legal counsel, an obvious slap at the prosecution. When Bill Wise called and told Hunter about this, he felt blindsided. The district attorney went on a Denver radio talk show the next morning and announced what the police planned to do. Three lawyers actually signed on to assist the police, two of them former prosecutors, one a former officer himself, and one the dean of the University of Denver Law School. All would work pro bono. In a statement to the media, Alex Hunter acknowledged this was "unusual in a criminal investigation," but drolly added, "Almost everything about this case is unusual."[23]

Shortly after the discovery of JonBenet Ramsey's body, Americans were turning to that new electronic back fence, the Internet, to discuss the details of the case and to share their opinions. By the summer of 1997, one Internet author had caught on with the public and had even drawn the attention of the police. Called Jameson and based in Hickory, North Carolina, this Web site had regularly been presenting information that the Boulder police had not yet made public and some facts that even they did not know about. The author's name, Sue Bennett, further intrigued police, since "Bennett" was John Ramsey's mother's maiden name. Hearing from her sources that Lou Smit had been steering an independent course in his investigation, Bennett contacted the investigator and shared with him her theory that JonBenet had been killed by someone who had entered her home while the family was out on Christmas evening and had hidden in the home's basement. Smit listened carefully and then directed Bennett to contact the Boulder police. Bennett was only one of the hundreds, even thousands, of people who had made the JonBenet Ramsey murder case a full-time preoccupation. I myself also received hundreds of letters and telephone calls from persons offering their opinions or offering their services to help with the investigation. Even though the lawyers for the Ramseys had agreed not to reveal the contents of the ransom note, the couple's continued advertising campaign gave out certain particulars. Rather than being angry at this, Alex Hunter hoped that this kind of pressure could lead to a genuine breakthrough in the case. There was also now a $500,000 reward being offered by one of the tabloid newspapers, and it was hoped this might also get someone to step forward with fresh and crucial information.

In mid-August the full autopsy report was made public. There were no crucial revelations in the material that had been withheld, most of it dealing with autopsy details. These included the fact that JonBenet's body was covered by a Colorado Avalanche hockey team sweatshirt after it was placed on the floor of the living room upstairs and that there was a sequined star on the front of her knit nightshirt. The news reporters were, in fact, becoming increasingly frustrated about how the case was standing still. Many were openly worried about being pulled from the assignment or even losing their jobs, since there was so little to report. Alex Hunter remained the lightning rod for the case. When a writer from *Vanity Fair* magazine in New York came to Boulder, she interviewed him for forty-five minutes and then sat in his office while he and his top people watched the televised coverage of Timothy McVeigh's conviction for the Oklahoma City bombing. After the group had broken up, Hunter continued to answer questions and talk for another hour and a half. Within a few days, the reporter wanted a follow-up session with Hunter and specifically told Suzanne Laurion, the district attorney's press aide, that she wanted certain answers clarified. Hunter balked when he heard the nature of the secondary questions, since, as he told Laurion, those comments had been "off the record." The second interview was never granted, particularly after Bill Wise and others heard that she was purportedly trying to dig up dirt on Hunter and his top people. The *Vanity Fair* writer refused Laurion's suggestion that she submit written questions to her boss. Hunter had also become very familiar with reporters from *Time* and *Newsweek*, the national newsmagazines. At times, these reporters sent him memos full of advice on how to handle the national media.

On Saturday, August 29, Hunter announced in a news release that he would not, after all, be making the trip the following week to the FBI conference in Quantico. Hunter had come to this conclusion when he was informed by Tom Wickman, a top police detective, that not all of the evidence had been forwarded to the bureau, another clear sign that the Boulder police did not wish to share their findings. Hunter reasoned that, like the local police, the FBI would not, then, be able to develop a complete and impartial overview of the case. Hunter had also made a phone call to a top bureau official who told the district attorney that the FBI was not prepared, with the limited evidence they had received, to say that there was enough against John and Patsy Ramsey to convict the couple, only enough to indict.

More and more of the Ramsey case seemed to have become a media event, a three-way game of chess being played out by the Ramseys, the police, and the prosecutors. Then, in the early morning hours of Sunday, August 31, the world was shocked to learn that Princess Diana of England and her wealthy boyfriend were killed on Saturday evening in an auto accident in Paris. This did more than distract the media's and the country's attention from the Ramsey case. The following Tuesday, *Larry King Live* on CNN featured a close look at the role the paparazzi—the freelance photographers often hired by the tabloid press—had played in causing these fatalities.

During his broadcast, Larry interrupted the dialogue by taking a call from Patsy Ramsey, who had been watching the show with her mother in the Atlanta area. Mrs. Ramsey attacked Tony Frost, editor of the *Globe*, the program's principal guest, who was sitting across from Larry in the studio. She condemned him for printing the stolen autopsy photos. "These tabloid photographers have ruined our lives," she said, adding that both the reporters and photographers were stalking her entire family. Patsy Ramsey added that she had been with her son, Burke, when he had seen a terrible headline in a tabloid, one that accused her husband and her of her daughter's murder. King tried to direct the dialogue toward the investigation, but Mrs. Ramsey told him that she couldn't talk about that. She credited John Ramsey with a "wonderful" idea, that photographers be forced to obtain a signed photo release form before publishing any photos of celebrities. Before running out of time, Larry King advised Mrs. Ramsey that "the only way this is going to stop is with you." Ironically, a producer from King's show had visited Boulder the previous week, attempting to line up an interview with John and Patsy Ramsey.

The afternoon of Patsy Ramsey's call to Larry King, an advance copy of the *Vanity Fair* article, entitled "Missing Innocence," began to circulate in Boulder. After reading the piece, Alex Hunter and Bill Wise immediately recognized that their work on the Ramsey case was in for some severe national criticism. The writer extensively quoted a Boulder police officer who bitterly attacked the district attorney and his top people, primarily for their dealings with the Ramsey defense team and, not too surprisingly, with the Boulder Police Department. The author also relied on secret police reports and openly attacked any notion that John and Patsy Ramsey could be innocent. In addition, the magazine published the full ransom note, the first time this had happened. Pete Hofstram's personal integrity was challenged, and the author claimed that he had been acting as though he was in awe of the Ramseys' defense attorneys. One unnamed police source called Lou Smit "a delusional old man."[24] Word about the article quickly spread throughout the Boulder and Denver media. That evening, one TV reporter read the entire ransom note on the air. The papers followed suit, with all attributing the note to the as-yet-unpublished *Vanity Fair* article. Many speculated on the identity of the article's key police source, making many of the top detectives, already in Quantico, very nervous. Hunter quickly recognized that the mainstream media would very likely follow suit and preconvict the Ramseys. This could badly complicate his seating an impartial jury from not just the Boulder and Denver areas, but anywhere in the country. The district attorney also knew that he was being personally attacked in the article, that his integrity, for the first time in his career, had been openly questioned. Still, much of the public's attention was focused thousands of miles to the east, to England, where preparations were underway for Princess Diana's funeral.

The FBI's briefing at Quantico, which I was later advised of, was very thorough and professional. Yet, especially in light of their not having all of the police evidence, it did not reveal any new avenues for the police to follow. The killer, in all probability, was someone who had access to the Ramsey home. The way the victim's body was found suggested that the assailant cared for his or her victim. The ransom note was written by an intelligent individual, but not a person experienced in criminal behavior. The note, like the child's body, pointed to someone very interested in diverting the investigators' attention. What "foreign faction" refers to itself as "small" and "foreign"? the FBI asked.[25] The note and all of the other activity seemed intended to establish the fact that a stranger did it. The experts did not rule out the possibility of someone from the outside killing JonBenet Ramsey, but they called that possibility "remote." The very long time taken by the assailant or assailants to write the note argued that there was no real fear of being discovered by some chance Ramsey holiday guest coming home late or, for that matter, by the family's dog, which no one knew had been sent across the street. Then there was the loud scream. This would have surely driven an outsider to leave the premises as soon as possible. The ligature around the victim's neck and wrist seemed staged. In fact, no one at the bureau had ever seen a child garroted after being fatally wounded with a blow to the head. However, this observation was merely statistical, so it could not be used as evidence. All of the materials used for the ransom note, the tape across the mouth, and the rope must have originated from within the Ramsey home. A stranger, who wanted to get in and out as quickly as possible, could never have known where to find these materials.

The Boulder police, during their portion of the dialogue, discussed the Ramseys' wanting to get out of town and back to Atlanta as quickly as possible. They admitted that their department bore much of the responsibility for John and Patsy Ramsey's not being quickly interrogated. The FBI countered that people react differently to a terrible trauma and cautioned against reading too much into what the Ramseys did. Still, the experts acknowledged, most of the time the parents of a victim are constantly on the phone to the police, demanding action. The Ramseys had not done this. The FBI wrapped up its presentation by exhorting the police to redouble their efforts. The long-awaited FBI conference had been helpful, but it, too, had proven inconclusive.[26] Afterward, Boulder detectives Steve Thomas and Ron Gosage traveled to Hickory, North Carolina, to visit the world's largest manufacturer of adhesive tape. The tape used had been manufactured only a month or so before the murder. Called Supertape, this product was distributed under the name Bron. This was significant since the tape the detectives had purchased in May of 1997 at McGuckin's Hardware store bore the brand names Supertape and Bron.

Alex Hunter now began to step back from the media and to take a new approach to solving this case. During an earlier meeting at the Denver airport, I had told the district attorney that there was a distinct possibility that JonBenet Ramsey had been accidentally killed by someone in her family and that the family had panicked and had decided to stage a cover-up to avoid anyone getting into terrible trouble. This represented a new hypothesis for him to fathom.

I was most interested in seeing everyone involved in the investigation take a step backward and start over. Alex Hunter was very receptive to this idea, and the Boulder police seemed to be improving their outlook. Since the police had brought their own three attorneys into the case, Hunter was finding Cdr. John Eller easier to deal with. Eller was obviously listening to his own counsel and had come to the conclusion that the police and district attorney's office did not have enough evidence to indict *and* convict the Ramseys. In late September, Police Chief Tom Koby announced that he was adding more detectives to the Ramsey investigation. There was plenty for them to do. Police detectives were recanvassing the Ramseys' old neighborhood and were searching for some play-mate of JonBenet's who could have exchanged clothing with her and, thus, be the source for the unidentified DNA found in her undergarments. Then, on September 29, the partially edited search warrants for the Ramsey house were made public, and the media interest was such that they quickly became "best-sellers." Much of what was disclosed had already been ferreted out by the media, who had speculated about what was still being held back. Alex Hunter had wondered how long it would be before someone leaked this information. The Ramsey defense team attacked the warrants for containing evidence of a more-recent scuffmark on the house's front door. This gained a good deal of attention until Arlene Beckworth, the family's former housekeeper, provided the explanation that sev-eral months before the crime a protective metal plate on the door jamb had fallen off, leaving the mark.

Boulder police chief Tom Koby and Alex Hunter enjoyed a good working relationship. In spite of John Eller's becoming more schooled on the legal difficulties facing the district attorney and whether he could arrest John and Patsy Ramsey, Hunter still felt that Eller needed to be replaced. He also knew that his own position, like those of Koby and Eller, was becoming precarious. In the first week of October, Hunter was asked to meet with Koby. The district attorney must have assumed that the first order of business would be the chief's decision to replace Eller. When Hunter got to Koby's office, he was astounded to hear a tape recording of a conversation between a tabloid reporter and a Boulder detective. Hunter had been friendly to the tabloid reporter and had confided in him, a mistake, it had turned out. The reporter told the detective about Hunter's feel-ings toward Eller and his need to be replaced and how Hunter had leaked information to his employer, the *Globe*.[27] After this meeting,

Koby told Eller that he was, indeed, replacing him with a highly organized, college-educated, veteran police administrator, Mark Beckner, a man who had come up through the Boulder police ranks. Under their new commander, the detectives were no longer going to decide what their assignments were, as they had previously been able to do. Eller was still going to be chief of the detective bureau, but his responsibilities were no longer going to include the Ramsey investigation. He would be retiring on February 28, 1998. A few days later Koby told Hunter that he was closing down the war room.

Alex Hunter was now beginning an offensive of his own. Working through a regional organization of Colorado prosecutors, he had formed a special task force to assist him in the Ramsey case. He was also meeting discreetly with big-time television producers, people who worked directly for Tom Brokaw at NBC and Larry King at CNN. To encourage his own staff, Hunter emphasized Pete Hofstram's excellent twenty-three-year career. Hofstram also had been bolstered by Eller's being replaced by Mark Beckner, and Hofstram was immediately communicating better with the police. Hunter was doing more than trying to put the *Vanity Fair* article and some other press blunders behind him. He was focusing on developing an experienced team to eventually take the Ramsey case through a successful prosecution. Denver district attorney Bob Grant was one member of his new regional prosecutors' team who kept pressing Hunter to think about adding attorneys to his team, veterans who had actually prosecuted a murder case like this one in court. Hunter was listening. He knew that, eventually, he would need this outside assistance, whether there was an arrest or the case was finally submitted to a grand jury.

As the weeks dragged into late fall, Chief Tom Koby continued to be a target of the police union. In November there was another vote of no confidence, and the union planned to follow up with a second vote the next month. Police referred to Koby as "dead man walking." This time Koby decided he'd had enough and announced that he would be resigning at the end of 1998. One of the unresolved disputes that Koby hoped to leave behind involved Det. Sgt. Larry Mason, who had been suspended by John Eller early in the year. The police union voted to reimburse Mason, but he never returned to his old job and eventually left the force, even though the Board of Police Commissioners voted in early 1998 to exonerate him. In early November, Lockheed Martin, the parent firm of Access Graphics, announced that it had sold the Boulder company and other local assets to General Electric for $2.8 billion in stock. John Ramsey would leave the firm, though he could stay on with Lockheed Martin for another half year. Shortly after this announcement, several attorneys representing Ramsey met with Hunter to discuss the fact that their client had lost a great deal of money in this transaction and that he would soon be unemployed. Hunter saw that this meeting was a veiled threat to sue the city of Boulder for their client's economic hardship. Hunter quickly dismissed the meeting.[28] Ramsey himself gave an occasional off-the-record interview to a reporter and was interviewed extensively by a University of Colorado journalism professor for a proposed British Broadcasting Corporation program that would be aired in 1998.

The police department's to-do list assembled during the FBI Quantico meeting, and subsequently reviewed when the investigation was reorganized, now became a top priority for investigators. Det. Carey Weinheimer traveled to St. Clair Shores, Michigan, to consult with Dr. Werner Spitz, a world-renowned forensic pathologist whom I had recommended. Dr. Spitz, upon seeing photos of the victim's damaged vagina and other autopsy photos, decided to travel to Boulder to conduct his own investigation, arriving there in mid-November. Dr. Spitz, who is also an old friend of mine, said that the vaginal damage must have occurred either shortly before or at the victim's time of death. He also said that the partially digested pineapple chunks indicated that JonBenet had eaten them an hour and a half prior to death, which meant that she had died around a half hour after midnight, given an 11:00 PM bedtime. Dr. Spitz was joined by Tom Faure, the coroner's chief investigator, and Weinheimer. The group studied the cellulose substance that was found in the victim's vagina and determined that it was consistent with the wood from the broken shard of the paintbrush handle used in the garroting. They also found that JonBenet had sustained a very powerful blow to the head, which, though it did not cause external bleeding, caused intracerebral bleeding that would quickly prove fatal. They could not determine if the head blow preceded the garroting with scientific certainty, though the head blow, in all probability, had come first. Since the head wound was fully developed, this meant that the victim had survived for a period of time. Dr. Spitz said that there had been no prior wounds to the vagina and that the cellulose dated from her time of death. Other experts later disagreed, saying that this damage had occurred much earlier that night. CBI investigators continued to wrestle with the weak and contaminated DNA samples taken from under the victim's fingernails, and determined these samples could not provide accurate findings. The list of unresolved issues continued to grow.

On December 1 a team of three attorneys who were defending John and Patsy Ramsey met with Alex Hunter to get a sense of where the case was and where the district attorney thought it would be going. Hunter took the occasion to urge the attorneys to have their clients come in for more interviews with the police. He added that the Ramseys' image was bound to be further tarnished if they did not agree to unconditional interviews. Patrick Burke, who was Patsy Ramsey's lawyer, complained about misinformation in the press, specifically that Burke Ramsey had not been interviewed when he had talked directly to the police once and to a child psychologist while the police watched a second time. During this tense meeting, Hunter also warned that pressure was mounting for the case to go to a grand jury. On December 5 Mark Beckner held a news conference to discuss the progress he felt was being made on the investigation. He was flanked by the seven detectives who were now working the case. Beckner said that when he'd taken this new job nine weeks earlier, there had been a list of seventy-two tasks that needed completing, and twenty-eight of those had already been accomplished. In response to a reporter's question, Beckner said that John and Patsy Ramsey were not suspects, but that they had been under "an umbrella of suspicion," as had many others who had come and passed under that umbrella. He added that the police wanted to ask the Ramseys more questions and that it was common police practice to reinterview individuals. Beckner also said that since he had been in his job, the Ramseys had cooperated with several requests.

The Christmas season of 1997 brought back poignant memories of JonBenet Ramsey and how the little girl had died. The First United Methodist Church of Boulder held a memorial service for JonBenet on December 14. The program "A Christmas Message from the Entire Ramsey Family" also appeared on a Web site that the Ramseys had established. In their message, the Ramseys had used the words "and hence," a phrase that had appeared in the ransom note. Several investigators, including Lou Smit, looked closely at that fact. Smit then received a letter from John Ramsey asking that four men be investigated closely as his daughter's possible murderer. Three were ex-employees of Access Graphics, and the fourth was Austin O'Rourke, the Santa Claus from the Ramsey Christmas party. A reporter from the *Rocky Mountain News* of Denver had found out about the Hi-Tec shoe print found in the dust on the floor of the wine cellar. A Ramsey defense lawyer wrote the reporter an impassioned letter asking the paper not to run the story. Alex Hunter, when told about this development, was also upset since this disclosure could directly interfere with the investigation. If the shoe print was significant, the person who had left it, with the shoe company's distinct logo, could then easily dispose of that pair of shoes. The paper ran the story. Many reporters were canvassing the Ramseys' neighborhood themselves, and a *Los Angeles Times* reporter was told by one woman that a police detective had specifically asked her about a stun gun. The reporter asked Bill Wise about this, and, because he had been out of the loop for many months, Wise knew nothing about it, calling the report "just another crazy rumor." This story broke on December 21, and the Ramseys' press aide was quick to claim that only an outsider could use a weapon so cruel on JonBenet.

As Christmas day itself approached, the city of Boulder was again rocked by a homicide. Susannah Chase, a twenty-three-year-old University of Colorado student from Connecticut, was found beaten into a coma late on the night of December 21. She was found in an alley behind her home and not far from Pasta Jay's

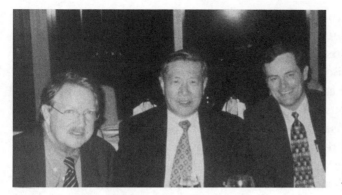

District Attorney Alex Hunter (left), Assistant District Attorney Michael Kane (right), and Dr. Lee (center) meeting.

restaurant, owned by the man who had taken the Ramsey family into his home less than a week after JonBenet Ramsey's murder. After lingering two days in critical condition, Chase, beaten almost beyond recognition by an assailant wielding a baseball bat, died. Chief Koby placed John Eller in charge of this investigation, and Eller reassigned detectives working on the Ramsey case to this latest murder. Alex Hunter was puzzled at Eller's appointment. As though on cue, he believed that Eller was already withholding evidence from Boulder County sheriff George Epp and a murderer was on the loose, one who posed a much greater danger to the citizens of Boulder. History repeats itself. The same mistakes were made in the investigation of the Chase murder as were made in the Ramsey case. Not until two years later, at the constant urging of Susannah Chase's parents, did the Boulder Police Department contact me and ask me to assist them in reconstructing the case. Unfortunately, this request came two years too late. During a meeting with the Boulder detectives working the case, I was apprised of the fact that the murder weapon was a baseball bat, which I was shown. This bat should have been publicized as soon as it was found, to generate information from the general public on the identity of its owner. Instead, due to orders from above, the bat was kept in an evidence room in the detective bureau—a secret. In addition, the victim's house keys were reported missing and could not be found. Detectives worked on the theory that most likely the assailant took those keys. But during my reexamination of her jacket, I found the keys in her pocket, where they'd been all the time. Thus, a timely opportunity to solve this crime was lost. This homicide remains unsolved today.

Meanwhile, Boulder detectives had asked their trio of lawyers to walk through the Ramsey house. When the police and attorneys arrived at the house, they realized that no one had a key to get in. A detective let himself into the house through a window, only to see security cameras recording every move. The embarrassed police confiscated the cameras and were later told that, too, was an illegal act.

As 1998 began, the Ramsey case, with its many players, seemed to be getting crazier by the moment. Sanford Lucas and his wife were still infuriated that Alex Hunter had denied them transcripts of their previous statements to the police, when the district attorney had gone along with giving the Ramseys their transcripts. Hunter, of course, was concerned that by giving them to Lucas, he would later be accused of tainting Lucas as a prosecution witness. Mr. and Mrs. Lucas even went to Colorado governor Roy Romer to ask to have Hunter replaced on the Ramsey case by a special prosecutor. The governor, after checking with prosecutors and police, decided to keep Hunter on. The disgruntled Lucases finally wrote a lengthy letter to the Boulder *Daily Camera*, which Bill Wise rebutted the same day. All of this simply served to distract from the actual investigation itself. On January 12 an article by Lawrence Schiller appeared in the *New Yorker* magazine that attempted to bring its readers up to date on the Ramsey case and why District Attorney Alex Hunter had not yet indicted John or Patsy Ramsey. Pete Hofstram thought that this would add fuel to the police notion that Hunter had been leaking news stories to the press. Hofstram, alert to the notion that Hunter was purportedly leaking police information, even took the unusual step of not showing his boss certain police information, insulating Hunter when and if those facts found their way into the media.[29]

Mark Beckner was proving a knowledgeable and professional police commander, one that Alex Hunter was learning to deal with on a regular basis. This was a huge improvement. John and Patsy Ramsey had, through their attorneys, rejected any further interviews with the police. Beckner tried to establish a direct line of communication with the couple, working through the Reverand Rol Hoverstock, pastor of Boulder's St. John's Church, where the Ramsey family had worshiped. Beckner had even offered to travel to Atlanta to question the Ramseys, an initiative they at first seemed receptive to, but one they later turned down. Police speculated that the couple's defense lawyers had advised against that meeting. Meanwhile, the prosecutors on Alex Hunter's special advisory committee were preparing him for the eventual convening of a grand jury. Bill Ritter, the Denver district attorney, and another member of that committee, suggested Michael Kane as the best grand jury specialist he had ever known. Kane, a former assistant prosecutor, lived in Chambersburg, Pennsylvania, about twenty-five miles west of Gettysburg, where he worked for the state department of revenue.

John Ramsey, meanwhile, was negotiating a new position for himself, a partnership with a Spanish software company that specialized in editing and composition work for TV. CNN was already a client. Ramsey became head of North American operations for Jaleo Technologies, responsible for its marketing and product development. Ramsey immediately began to attract other high-caliber executives to Jaleo. The Ramsey family traveled to Spain as part of these negotiations, and a reporter from a tabloid newspaper published a story saying that the family had fled to Spain since it did not have an extradition treaty with the United States. Lockheed Martin bought the Ramsey house for $650,000, as part of its employment contract with John Ramsey. They then sold the house to a limited-liability partnership headed by friends of the Ramseys. Any profits from its ultimate sale were to go to a charity named for JonBenet. As per their agreement with the police, John and Patsy Ramsey turned over a good deal of clothing to investigators. The red-and-black checkered jacket worn by Patsy on Christmas night was one item that detectives were planning to look at very closely, because of the red and black fibers found attached to the duct tape over JonBenet's mouth. This was sent to the CBI for laboratory analysis.

In early February of 1998 I received a phone call while I was in San Francisco from Carol McKinley, whom I had met several years earlier. She had formerly been a Denver radio newsperson and now worked for Fox News. Carol asked what I thought the chances were of the Ramsey case ever being solved, and I replied that on a scale of one to ten, I gave it a two. Carol then jumped on a plane to San Francisco and taped my comments in person. Alex Hunter wanted me to come back to meet with the detectives one more time to try to get the investigation moving forward again. On February 13 I met with Hunter, Mark Beckner, Lou Smit, Trip DeMuth, and police detectives Wickman and Trujillo. We discussed the case for six hours. Afterward, we held a press briefing. I now gave the case a fifty-fifty chance of being solved. Alex Hunter was already prepared to advise the media that I was there to talk with the police and not for his staff. In his remarks, he criticized John and Patsy Ramsey as being uncooperative with the police, particularly about consenting to more interviews. This was the first time that the district attorney had openly criticized JonBenet's parents. Hunter also seemed gratified that there was not the usual glut of reporters and photographers from around the country. Perhaps the fervent national interest in the case was abating.

Mark Beckner's excellent work was not going unnoticed. In late February news stories revealed he was being appointed chief of the Boulder Police Detective Bureau. At about the same time, John Eller retired and drove off to Florida, his home state. In the first week of March, Beckner began to pressure the district attorney's staff, Pete Hofstram in particular, for the convening of a grand jury. On March 12 the Boulder police formally asked for a grand jury to handle the Ramsey case. Hofstram told Beckner that it would take at least six months after the district attorney's office was given the files to get up to speed. Hofstram knew that the police didn't have enough for a conviction and seemed to be stalling for time. Bob Grant, who had been acting as a spokesman for Hunter, went on television and said that a month would be adequate. Hunter also disagreed with Hofstram's time estimate. The district attorney's office had to explain to Beckner that, once the grand jury got the case, matters would then be out of the hands of the police and the district attorney's office. The incumbent Boulder grand jury's term was due to expire on May

30. District Judge Joseph Bellipanni set April 22 as the date when the court would begin impaneling a new grand jury, chosen from 150 ordinary citizens summoned for this duty. Alex Hunter was particularly worried over whether the court could find twelve citizens and five alternates who were unbiased enough to sit in judgment on this case. Public opinion polls showed that, across the nation, a large majority of Americans who said they knew about the case thought that a Ramsey family member was responsible for the crime.

The three attorneys advising the Boulder police suggested to their clients that they create a multimedia presentation of the investigation when they turned the case over to the district attorney's office in the next month or so. This appealed to the detectives, in particular, who had been frustrated by their inability to communicate directly what they felt was damaging evidence against the Ramseys. Alex Hunter announced to his staff on April 9 that he was asking Michael Kane to join him for the grand jury that surely lay ahead. A few days later Hunter met with Judge Bellipanni and showed him the lengthy jury questionnaire used for seating the Oklahoma City bombing proceedings. Judge Bellipanni resisted going more than one page, but relented to allow a second page, in light of the possibility of the jurors' hearing about the JonBenet Ramsey case. Then, on April 15, Ramsey defense lawyer Bryan Morgan hand-delivered a two-page letter from John Ramsey to Hunter. In it, Ramsey promised to make himself; his wife; his son, Burke; and friends and business associates available for interviews to the district attorney's office, once they had control of the case. The Boulder police were not to be anywhere near these sessions. Hunter was impressed and demanded a taping of these interviews, which Morgan initially refused. When Hunter held his ground, Morgan relented, indicating that John Ramsey was now calling the shots. Hunter told Beckner about all of this. Both men must have seen that Ramsey might be attempting to avoid a grand jury appearance.

On April 22, Hunter and Pete Hofstram appeared before Judge Bellipanni and began questioning the 150 prospective jurors assembled there. The JonBenet case was the obvious focus of many of their questions, sort of like an eight-hundred-pound gorilla sitting in the corner of the room. The national media had returned in force and sat in the gallery. At the end of the day, Judge Bellipanni selected twelve grand jurors, four men and eight women, and five alternates, one man and four women. Most came from Boulder or Longmont.

Sanford Lucas still wanted copies of his previous statements. He met with Mark Beckner and was refused, though Beckner relented a little and promised that Lucas could read copies while he was at police headquarters. Lucas refused and left, infuriated. He then let it be known that he was no longer cooperating in the case in any way. Det. Linda Arndt represented a similar problem. Arndt told Det. Steve Thomas that she had not recorded any notes and that she had no memory of that entire morning, December 26. Though still on the force, Arndt was suing the department for what she considered defamation of her professional character. Thomas pleaded with Arndt, to no avail, and then determined that he would have to report her to his superiors as uncooperative.[30] Meanwhile, Michael Kane had reported for duty. Pete Hofstram, due to his usual heavy case-load, was pleased to be able to greet him. Kane's reputation as a hard-nosed and strictly business prosecutor had preceded him. Kane was very clear in his advice to Hunter about dealing with the media: Don't. Keep your mouth shut. Hunter listened attentively and then withdrew behind a wall of silence. The battle lines for the grand jury were rapidly forming. Meanwhile, the Boulder detectives continued to throw themselves into preparing their presentation. They were bolstered by the FBI's and CBI's findings on the fibers taken from Patsy Ramsey's checkered jacket. They were consistent, although the fibers still could have come from a similar material.

Barry Scheck and I traveled to Boulder on Sunday, May 31, to attend the investigators' prehearing presentation. Bill Wise picked us up at the Denver airport. I would be going on to Taiwan to assist in a mass-murder case. A mayor and a city councilman and their body-guards had all been gunned down at the mayor's residence. From there I was going to the Philippines to lecture to police and at a medical school. Barry Scheck and I had never seen the interior of the Ramsey house, and we then toured the big, empty structure. We started our inspection from the house's exterior. I tried to lift the iron grate above the train-room window and to climb down into the window well, which I was barely able to do. I looked up at Barry and a couple of other investigators, and I joked that they couldn't make it through the window because of their size and body shapes. Inside, we were all struck by how dark the interior of the house was and that a person, even one who had studied the layout of the house, would have had trouble getting around. For instance, the door to the basement was very awkward to open, and it was difficult to find a light switch, which, illogically, was located on the opposite wall. I took out my magnifying glass and studied the basement walls and floor. I photographed the rooms against a scale. I stood at the door to the wine cellar and first looked in very quickly, as Sanford Lucas had reported he'd done. The room was very dark. There was a foot-thick concrete wall immediately to my right, and I had to turn my head to the left to look into the room. There was a bare lightbulb immediately outside the doorway, and it did not shine into the space. If one weren't looking down, one might miss seeing a white blanket on the floor and the little girl's hands protruding out toward the observer. After the tour, we all went back to the Justice Center for a briefing, and later Barry and I were invited to Alex Hunter's home for a dinner, an unobstructed view of the Flatirons, and some pleasant conversation about forensic science and my many ventures of travel around the world.

We have learned that the day prior to my visit to Alex Hunter's home, he had been working in his backyard when his son answered the phone. The nine-year-old was incredulous when the caller said he was John Ramsey. Mrs. Hunter was equally skeptical. When Alex got on the line, he had to quickly advise Ramsey that ethical canons prevented him from talking to him until and if Ramsey's lawyers gave their assent. Hunter also explained that his short conversation with Mrs. Ramsey in February of 1997 had been one-way, his merely listening to her compliments on what he had said. Ramsey then tried to contact his lawyers and, unsuccessful, flew the next day to Denver. It was obvious that Ramsey very much wanted to cooperate with Hunter, once he formally got the case. Meanwhile, a reporter from the *Globe* called Hunter two days later and repeated the gist of that phone conversation. Hunter told the reporter that he was now wondering if his phone was tapped, which was all the confirmation the reporter needed. Over Hunter's protests, the paper ran the story. Meanwhile, Pete Hofstram was working hard to set up ground rules for questioning Burke Ramsey. The boy's attorney was proving most cooperative, even allowing anyone of Hofstram's choosing to interview Burke. The lawyer said there would be no other conditions, either. The two set June 10 as a target date, and Hofstram would even travel to Atlanta to see that everything went smoothly.

On Monday morning, June 1, Barry Scheck and I accompanied Alex Hunter into the Coors Events Center on the University of Colorado campus. A large knot of media photographers, correspondents, and TV reporters crowded outside the entrance, and several shouted questions to Hunter, who answered only that he was there to listen. The Boulder Police Department gave a final presentation of their evidence in the JonBenet Ramsey murder case. The detectives chose a tiered lecture hall to do this. The district attorney's lawyers and investigators, agents from the FBI's Child Abduction and Serial Killer Unit, investigators and laboratory scientists from the CBI, and others who had worked on the case sat in the room's rising seats. Typical for this investigation, all present had to endure a stifling hot atmosphere since the building's air-conditioning unit had malfunctioned. Every ninety minutes, there was a break. All of us paid close attention to the complicated array of facts, presented with Powerpoint slides, photos, and charts, as the Boulder police made their case. I took notes as Barry Scheck typed into a laptop. Specifics from the autopsy were followed by physical evidence, such as the flashlight found on the Ramseys' kitchen counter. This was a potential murder weapon, we were told, although there were no traces of blood or other tissues found on it. The investigators acknowledged that the trace amounts of foreign DNA evidence taken from under the victim's fingernails were weak, yet their presentation excluded the Ramseys and other individuals who had been investigated based on this DNA.

During a playback of Patsy Ramsey's 911 call, some of us were surprised that JonBenet's mother did not sound more distraught.

During the discussion of the black fibers found on the duct tape and how they seemed to match the jacket worn by Mrs. Ramsey on Christmas night, I worried that some of the investigators had confused the term "microscopically similar" with a "scientific match." Also, the fibers could have originally gotten onto the blanket by a simple secondary transfer while a mother kissed her child goodnight and then later were transferred from the blanket to the tape. The ransom note was studied, and the fine-line Sharpie pen used to write it was established as from the Ramsey house. In the afternoon, I was forced to ask about information about pineapple, a tea cup and water glass on the table, and the origin of the panties she wore, material that I had told the detectives was needed a year earlier but had never been produced. This was during a question-answer session. Toward the end of the day, Det. Steve Thomas presented sixteen arguments on why the case should go to a grand jury. Some of these seemed frivolous, such as the December 25 date placed on their daughter's headstone by her parents. Others were compelling, such as John and Patsy Ramsey's behavior when the police arrived and, then, throughout the day. At the conclusion of the day-long presentation, Alex Hunter first met with his staff and the FBI. He also conferred at length with Barry Scheck and me. Hunter said he planned to have his office interview John and Patsy Ramsey. After this meeting, the district attorney went outside and told the media that he thought taking the case to a grand jury was most likely a logical next step, but that he still had to make that determination. As with so many elements in this case, the day's presentation seemed to breed more doubts than facts.

The Boulder police began the process of turning over the hundreds of volumes of their investigative records and the thousands of items of the case's evidence to Alex Hunter's office. Mark Beckner urged that the district attorney's office subpoena John and Patsy Ramsey's credit card and phone records, prior to the couple's being interviewed again. These could refute the couple's saying, as they had in their interviews the previous April, that they had never purchased duct tape or cord. Hunter's staff refused, since it would mean delaying the next Ramsey interviews.

Things went smoothly when police reinterviewed Burke Ramsey for three days in Atlanta. Dan Schuler, a Colorado police officer known for his abilities in dealing with children, asked the questions while Pete Hofstram and a Ramsey attorney watched the two-hour sessions from an adjoining room and Patsy Ramsey waited in a local district attorney's office elsewhere in the building. Schuler asked Burke about what had occurred when the family had returned home from the Lucases' house on Christmas night. Had he eaten any pineapple? Burke said he didn't remember. The next morning, Burke had heard voices but had stayed in bed, pretending to be asleep, until his father woke him up to go to the Lucases' house. Schuler asked if JonBenet had ever made her parents very angry at her. Burke didn't think so. He also did not remember his sister causing her own death accidentally. Det. Jane Harmer was in a hotel room in Atlanta, where each evening she reviewed the day's tapes, and Hofstram also sent tapes each night to Boulder, where Michael Kane and other investigators studied them. Harmer and the others then called Schuler, suggesting lines of questioning for the following day. The six hours of questioning did not produce anything significant for the investigation. There was also no answer concerning the background voice on the 911 tape. The interviews did indicate, however, that John and Patsy Ramsey were determined to cooperate, now that Alex Hunter's office had the case.

On Monday, June 22, Michael Kane and Trip DeMuth, each with his own investigator, began interviewing John and Patsy Ramsey in separate rooms in Broomfield, not far from Boulder, a location selected since its small airport could unobtrusively accommodate the Ramseys' private jet. Both John and Patsy Ramsey would have an attorney and an investigator present during the questioning. One or two alert reporters suspected that these new interrogations were imminent, but none knew for sure. The Boulder police were kept out of the loop, though Michael Kane had been able to earn the confidence of several key detectives. Both Kane and DeMuth contacted me for advice on what to ask their respective subjects, and I counseled them to look for as many specifics as possible and to use the facts that the Ramseys did not know were established, such as the undigested pineapple chunks in their daughter's upper intestine and the tea cup and water glass, as well as facts on the duct tape and rope. The district attorney's two attorneys also consulted the FBI, the CBI, and Boulder police detectives. The interviews lasted until Thursday evening, June 25, and these sessions also produced nothing important. During her twenty hours of questioning, Patsy Ramsey surprised her interrogators with her toughness, which came out when she was accused of lying to them. When told there was physical evidence that contradicted what she had said, Mrs. Ramsey demanded to see it. For his part, John Ramsey implicated others, such as Austin O'Rourke, who had played Santa Claus for the family's Christmas party and whom JonBenet would have trusted. Ramsey said that O'Rourke could have fed his daughter the pineapple chunks. Besides, O'Rourke was broke, Santa's accuser claimed. Ramsey also observed that Sanford Lucas, once his best friend, was an experienced sailor and could have purchased the cord and duct tape. Also, Renee Lucas was from California, where women made it a practice to carry a stun gun for their own protection. Like Burke Ramsey's interviews, these open-ended sessions produced no direct answers to those unananswered issues.[31]

Following the interviews, Alex Hunter met with his staff. Michael Kane, in particular, was certain that the case now had to go to a grand jury, and Hunter agreed. Lou Smit, who had assisted Kane with the John Ramsey interviews, informed Hunter that his wife had experienced a recurrence of cancer and that he would be forced to cut his exhaustive schedule back to twenty hours a week so he could spend more time with her. Smit still felt that the murder had probably been committed by an intruder. As reporters got wind that the Ramsey interviews were taking place, there was a rush to put specifics onto the airwaves and into print. Very little actually came out. The following week, *Newsweek* carried an exchange between Lou Smit and John Ramsey in which Mr. Ramsey denied that his daughter had died in some sort of domestic accident. "Look, somebody bashed my daughter's head in. Somebody strangled her. It wasn't any accident." This information could have come from either the district attorney's office or the police, whose people watched tapes of the interviews each evening. On June 23, Mark Beckner was named to replace Tom Koby as chief of the Boulder Police Department. Koby worked for a short while in the city manager's office and then retired. After Koby's departure, Alex Hunter praised his friend's service to Boulder. In his own ranks, Hunter was faced with the fact that Pete Hofstram did not feel that there was enough evidence against John and Patsy Ramsey to take the case to a grand jury and asked to be allowed to go back to his other duties. Hunter had to respect his chief trial lawyer's decision. Instead, of course, Hunter had Michael Kane, his grand jury specialist, working for him.

Though rumors circulated about the Ramsey case going to a grand jury, Alex Hunter did not want to announce publicly his decision while John and Patsy Ramsey were proving cooperative. However, when Hal Haddon, one of the Ramseys' principal attorneys, released a statement claiming his clients had been quietly cooperating with the district attorney's office for eighteen months, Alex Hunter called the media to deny this claim. Many wondered if the Ramseys were cooperating now both to avoid a grand jury and to rehabilitate their reputations. And investigators began to follow up on what John Ramsey had said about Austin O'Rourke. The retired college professor and his wife were then making their final preparations to move to Massachusetts. They were called in to talk to Lou Smit and Dan Schuler, the detective who had interviewed Burke Ramsey. The two questioned the couple for seven hours, particularly about their leaving the country to fly to Spain within ten days of the murder. In making the trip, O'Rourke had been forced to carry heavy bags throughout several airports when his wife and he had changed planes. This went to the question about whether he was still physically able to commit the murder and to make his escape. Both investigators felt that Mr. and Mrs. O'Rourke needed further attention.

Boulder police detective Steve Thomas, who had been one of the lead investigators of the case, was in failing health. All of the hours he'd been putting into the case and the personal stress had taken their toll. Still only thirty-seven, Thomas had been suffering from a thyroid problem and sleep deprivation. On August 6, over Mark Beckner's protests, Thomas published a long and detailed letter of resignation. In this eight-page document, he attacked Alex Hunter for the way he'd handled the Ramsey case. He specifically criticized Hunter for not calling for a grand jury early in the case, so that those who refused to cooperate would be compelled to testify while everyone's memory of the events was much fresher. Thomas was particularly bitter about the way the case had been tried in the media and how his department had been depicted as incompetent. He said that, in his opinion, the killer of JonBenet Ramsey would never be brought to justice, at least not in this lifetime.[32]

The Thomas letter proved another bombshell. Alex Hunter, its principal target, had used this lull in the investigation to take his family to Alaska for a vacation, his first in the eighteen months since he'd returned from vacation in January of 1997. Even Colorado governor Roy Romer began hearing about what Thomas had to say, and the feedback was both angry and from respected friends. There was talk about the governor's appointing a special prosecutor, in effect replacing Hunter. Finally, Beckner publicly disagreed with Thomas's assertion that the case could not be successfully concluded. Still, the letter had seemed to touch a public nerve. Many citizens were feeling the same frustrations as Steve Thomas. Governor Romer contacted Bob Grant of the metropolitan district attorney's committee that had been assisting Hunter. Alex Hunter called in from Alaska on the following Saturday, and, after listening to Thomas's letter, he immediately truncated his vacation and made plans to return to Boulder. Hunter was particularly worried that the letter could become cannon fodder for a shrewd defense attorney in a trial. The fact that Detective Thomas had long been identified as a key investigator gave his bitter criticism credibility.

On Wednesday, August 12, Alex Hunter and his top people met with Bob Grant and the metropolitan district attorneys who had been advising Hunter. Grant and his group said they supported Hunter's actions and later, after meeting alone with Hunter, called Governor Romer. They told Romer that the group felt that Michael Kane could use some extra help and recommended Al LaCabe, a former police officer and a prosecutor in the US attorney's office in Denver, who, it turned out, could not be spared by his office. Grant also advised the governor that Hunter had been planning to send the case to the grand jury that was convening on September 15. Romer then decided to make that announcement himself later that afternoon, along with the metro district attorneys, who stood behind the governor at his news conference. Hunter and Wise returned to Boulder as Governor Romer stepped before the media and said that he had ruled out the appointment of a special prosecutor for the case. As part of their discussions with Grant and the district attorneys' committee, Hunter agreed that Pete Hofstram and any others in his office who did not totally support the grand jury would have nothing further to do with the Ramsey investigation. Later in August, Sanford and Renee Lucas wrote a letter to the press agreeing with Steve Thomas. Lucas, refusing to cooperate with the district attorney's office, was still smoldering over his inability to obtain a transcript of what he had previously told the police, and he'd already heard that John Ramsey was actively trying to implicate his wife and himself in JonBenet's murder. This could all combine to have Lucas indicted for perjury or worse.

Since the US attorney in Denver was understaffed and could not spare Al LaCabe, his top gun, Alex Hunter then decided to sign on two other prosecutors to assist Michael Kane who would be provided by members of the metro district attorney's organization. Bob Grant turned over his chief trial deputy, Bruce Levin, who was very experienced and was known for his excellent courtroom skills. Bill Ritter, another one of the metro district attorneys, recommended Mitch Morrissey from his staff. Hunter wondered whether these two attorneys were going to be able to master all of the complex evidence and facts of a case that had been investigated for more than twenty months in just the three weeks until the grand jury convened. Levin and Morrissey both had access to Tom Wickman, the Boulder police detective who was now serving as a key investigator for the grand jury, as well as other attorneys in the district attorney's office. Still, neither of the newcomers had attended the final police presentation of evidence. This seeming weakness, though, could prove a strong point since the two prosecutors would be seeing everything with fresh eyes. Michael Kane had already shown why he enjoyed such an excellent reputation. He worked on the case from dawn until late at night, taking only a few minutes off each day to run three miles. Kane met with Alex Hunter each day to apprise him of his progress. Hunter knew that if there was any disagreement between Kane and himself, the case was now in Kane's hands, and he would be the one making the calls.

On Sunday, September 13, Michael Kane, Bruce Levin, and Boulder detective Jane Harmer traveled to Arlene Beckworth's home in Fort Lupton to show the Ramseys' former housekeeper a volume of crime scene photos. The trio was particularly interested in photos of JonBenet's bedroom. There were two decorative curtains behind the victim's bed, and one of them had been untied and was hanging down behind the bed when police investigated the room. Beckworth agreed that this was extraordinary, but had no explanation as to why the curtain hung down that way. Could the child have pulled the curtain loose trying to hide behind it or protect herself from someone? Nobody knew. Police also had photographed a number of the child's hair ties that were scattered around on the floor at the foot of the bed. This, too, was unusual. The ties usually sat in a basket in the child's bathroom. Beckworth was then shown an open drawer in JonBenet's dresser, and she confirmed that was where her underpants were kept. Beckworth had not been asked any of these questions before. Beckworth was then shown photos of JonBenet's bed covered by a comforter and then of her white thermal blanket, which had urine and brownish stains on it. She then looked at a photo of the interior of the clothes dryer outside the child's bedroom and recognized the pink-and-white checkered sheets in it since she had put those on JonBenet's bed on December 23, the last time she'd made up the bed. Another photo showed JonBenet's bed had her *Beauty and the Beast* sheets covering it. Beckworth was unable positively to identify the bowl that had contained the chunks of pineapple, though she said it was like the ones she remembered. Finally, she was shown a photo of the Bible from John Ramsey's bedroom desk, opened, as usual, to Psalm 118. Then she began to weep, and Michael Kane consoled her.

THE JONBENET RAMSEY GRAND JURY PROBE

At around 8:00 AM on Tuesday, September 15, the twelve grand jurors and their four alternates began arriving at the Boulder Justice Center to begin their deliberations. The media had been provided with their names, and each could see his or her driver's license photo on the front page of the Boulder paper, the *Daily Camera*. Reporters and television and newspaper photographers had returned to Boulder in droves, and some called out greetings to the grand jurors who were escorted by a Boulder County sheriff as they walked toward the building's entrance. Police soon moved the media farther back to prevent any more communication with the grand jurors. When Alex Hunter arrived, the only comment he made to the press was "It's a beautiful day." Since the grand jury proceedings were secret, even the windows to courtroom L on the building's second floor, where the proceedings were initially convened, were covered by paper preventing any exposure to the outside world.

After an opening day of introduction, Michael Kane quickly began to present his case in a classic, timeline sequence of events. He started with the 5:52 AM, 911 phone call from Patsy Ramsey to the Boulder Police Department and moved forward from that instant. Det. Linda Arndt was one of his first witnesses, and she testified about being left alone in that large house for more than two hours without anyone heeding her calls for backup. This, of course, did not please Kane, since Arndt was essentially criticizing the case's investigation. Yet there wasn't much Kane could do about critical testimony since so many of the facts that followed spoke for themselves. All of the key police participants in the case's opening hours were called the first week. The following week the proceedings were moved down to the Justice Center's first floor, to courtroom E. Under Kane's direction, things continued to move along in an efficient manner. While all of this was going on inside the court of legal opinion, Lou Smit, the district attorney's investigator, wrote a letter to Alex Hunter resigning from the case and stating that he thought that John and Patsy Ramsey were being unjustly persecuted. Though Smit originally intended for his letter to be private, he gave in and provided a copy to a reporter, and the letter was soon transmitted to hundreds of news outlets by the Associated Press. Then ABC's *20/20* did a one-hour program on the Ramsey case, using the Smit letter and an interview with Steve Thomas, who spent most of his time explaining why he had resigned from the Boulder Police Department. However, none of this should have found its way into the grand jury room, since prosecutors routinely advised the jurors not to read about the case in the papers or to watch or listen to anything about it on television or radio. The grand jurors were to base their judgments solely on what was presented to them in the courtroom.

Alex Hunter, of course, attended all of the grand jury's sessions. Under Michael Kane's guidance, the process continued to move along smoothly, though at a deliberate pace. By October 27, it had convened only ten times and had taken a ten-day break. Two days later, the grand jurors spent the morning touring the Ramseys' former house and property. One man seemed very interested in the strength of the house's drainpipes and whether or not they might support the weight of an intruder. Each carried a pad of paper and a pen. The large house was now empty, and it seemed difficult to correlate the rooms with the crime scene photos. The grand jurors then returned to the Justice Center, and the proceedings continued to move forward.

The grand jury completed its deliberations in early October 1999, thirteen months after it was originally convened, without ever calling John or Patsy Ramsey to testify. Before the jury reached a verdict, Alex Hunter called me and asked that the two of us meet to spend a weekend going over all of the evidence developed in the grand jury room and elsewhere. Alex invited me to come to stay at his house, and I arrived in Boulder on October 8. I knew why it was vital to Alex that the two of us get together and pore over all the details in this highly complex case. He needed to be absolutely sure in his own mind that the next step that he took was, to the best of his ability, the right one. The two of us worked sixteen-hour days reviewing all of the case's evidence and statements. Late on the final day of my visit, I looked Alex Hunter straight in the eye and told him that if he did what I thought he would be doing, he would be destroying his career. After I boarded my return flight to Connecticut, I knew in my heart what this conscientious and valiant man was going to do. This was further confirmed for me on October 12, after Michael Kane came to my office in Meriden and we also reviewed the case for many hours. Finally, two days later, Alex Hunter announced to the world that "I and my prosecution task force believe we do not have sufficient evidence to [file] charges against anyone." This announcement caused a firestorm, and the Boulder prosecutor was widely criticized for his decision. This, to me, seemed extremely unfair. All of this case finally boiled down to the fact that the prosecution did not have nearly enough evidence to convict anyone of JonBenet's death, beyond a reasonable doubt.

Alex Hunter also must have known that, with his deciding against an indictment, he was ending his twenty-eight-year career as a prosecutor. In March of 2000, Hunter made it official by announcing he was not going to seek an eighth term as Boulder County's district attorney, ending twenty-eight years of service. Shortly afterward, Bill Wise announced he was leaving the district attorney's office, ending his long career. And that is exactly where the JonBenet Ramsey murder case has stood since then. Alex Hunter, Bill Wise, Mike Kane, and many others all did their utmost. The case's outcome reflects what our American system of justice is based upon, that a defendant must be considered innocent until proven guilty beyond a reasonable doubt.

THE SUMMARY

This has been a very lengthy chapter, and many of my observations, such as the contrived nature of the ransom note, have been presented as part of the case's investigation. I related this information since so many of the facts of the JonBenet Ramsey case were apparent to investigators at the time of their discovery. No one I've ever spoken with had ever seen or even heard about a ransom note like this one. The FBI experts who first looked at this text simply shook their heads in disbelief. I also do not want to belabor the obvious in my concluding comments on this case, but I must mention a few salient facts. From the very first moment a uniformed officer stepped into the Ramsey house early on the morning of December 26, the Boulder Police Department began making critical mistakes. A thorough search of those premises that dawn should have uncovered the little girl's corpse lying in the dark room off of the basement. Then no one would have been allowed to contaminate the crime scene by moving the body upstairs. Many more experienced homicide investigators and forensic scientists should have immediately been called to the case, instead of asking one detective to ride herd on a dozen or so distraught adults. The overtures of help from the FBI and other experienced investigative and forensic experts should not have been rebuffed by the Boulder detective commander. These are all very basic mistakes, the kind that doomed this investigation to failure.

As tensions mounted between the Boulder police and the district attorney's office, both organizations should have simultaneously recognized the disastrous consequences of this tribal warfare and brought it all to a quick end. Abraham Lincoln said it well: "A house divided against itself cannot stand." This blood feud, which distracted one and all from the task of solving this case, was only exacerbated by the overriding attention paid to the case by the media and the public. Leadership should have demanded and established a gag order ensuring no personnel talking to the media, except a designated official. This should have been for one and all. No special treatment for anyone, and the professional release of information to the media and the public only when and if it was warranted. More water under the bridge. More irreparable mistakes.

Most recently, an attorney for John and Patsy Ramsey has come forward to criticize the lack of investigation on the source for the second DNA traces found in the underpants worn by JonBenet. This was, according to this attorney, an example of the tunnel vision that investigators applied in this case. The underpants worn by JonBenet were an adult size 7. Where this underwear came from is still a mystery. Boulder detectives were able to find that this type of underwear were sold only in Bloomingdale's and manufactured in Asia.

Finally, what do I feel really happened to cause the death of Jon-Benet Ramsey? I do not know. I think that it is quite possible that some kind of horrific domestic accident may have occurred involving this extremely talented and attractive little girl. Perhaps she fell or was even pushed down that narrow staircase that led from her bedroom to the kitchen and struck her head against an object, such as a banister. Perhaps it was in some rough horseplay with someone. Perhaps this tragedy occurred in the course of an argument turned violent, or was the act of a sexual predator in Boulder. But who really knows? Unfortunately, the mishandling of the crime scene and the lack of physical evidence have severely impeded the chances of ever solving this case. Only one or two people really know the facts, and there is the strong probability that these individuals will never step forward and say what happened during the cold and dark hours after Christmas of 1996. I find this all very sad.

CHAPTER FOUR

THE LISA PENG CASE

ADULTERY AND DEATH

Instead of telling you there are no problems in this country and painting a rosy picture . . . about our society and your future, I am going to tell you the reality and the facts.

—Dr. Henry C. Lee
Commencement Address at
the University of New Haven, May 27, 1995

Most Americans know that this country's justice system is imperfect. To paraphrase the British statesman Sir Winston Churchill, I have found the American justice system to be full of pitfalls, complexities, and even some contradictions, but our criminal justice system is still as good as any that can be found throughout human history. Granting the presumption of innocence of the accused in a criminal proceeding, until and unless proven guilty in a court of law, is only one reason that many criminal prosecutions have come to conclusions that, by their nature, do not satisfy any of the parties to a crime. Upon this cornerstone, many other rules of evidence for criminal proceedings have been built as a result of the courts' decisions into this system, case by case. These rulings apply to many of the modern and sophisticated scientific advances set in place in the last century. It is permissible, for instance, for the police to use a polygraph to test whether or not a suspect is deceptive, but the results of that test, commonly referred to as a lie detector test, are not later admissible in a court of law. The famous *Frye* ruling that barred the introducing into evidence of polygraph results due to their inherent unreliability has led to a great deal of complexity in introducing new scientific evidence into our legal system.

In 1963 at the age of twenty-five, I left my job as the youngest captain on the Taipei police force and later came to the United States. I was ambitious and had savored success in my years on the police force in Taiwan. In the summer of 1960, while on duty, I met a beautiful young college student at police headquarters, and that encounter changed my life forever. Soon we fell in love, and this bright young lady became my wife, Margaret. Three years later, Margaret and I decided to make a new life for ourselves in the United States, because we both knew that we had so much to learn and that the American educational system was far superior to many others in the world. At that time, America was also the land of opportunity, and for me it was exactly where I wanted to make forensic science my career. Thus, with just about fifty dollars in our pockets, the two of us got off of a plane from Malaysia and headed for New York City. Neither Margaret nor I could speak much English, so those first few months were quite an adventure in survival. If you happen to have had dinner at The Shanghai, a Chinese restaurant at Forty-third Street and Third Avenue in New York City during that time span, I might have been your waiter. Or I might have been your Kung Fu teacher, if, at that time, you studied karate or self-defense. But the two of us somehow survived and prospered, so neither Margaret nor I have ever really looked back with any regrets. I still tell people wherever I travel around the globe that this is the best country in the

world. As long as you have a dream, and you worked hard toward`
fulfilling your dream, your dream will someday become a reality.

I have related a little about my formative years in Taiwan and our
coming to America because the individuals who are at the center of
this case also had a Chinese background. The stabbing death of
twenty-five-year-old Ranbing "Jennifer" Ji on August 18, 1993, along
with the suffocation of her five-month-old son, Kevin Ji, in their
Mission Viejo, California, apartment, directly implicated individuals
who had also come to this country to fulfill their dreams. Li-Yun
"Lisa" Peng and her businessman husband, Tseng Jyi "Jimi" Peng,
instantly became prime suspects in these terrible crimes, since Jennifer Ji was Mr. Peng's mistress, and Kevin was his illegitimate son. I
should mention here that Margaret and I have been happily married
for more than forty years and are the proud parents of two grown
children.

The Peng case eventually led to three separate trials. I first heard
about these crimes when Margaret Kuo, an excellent forensic scientist and the supervising criminalist in the Orange County Sheriff's
Department Forensic Laboratory, an old friend of mine, contacted
me and asked for my interpretation of the case and crime scene.
Years later and many thousands of miles away, Lisa Peng's family
attorney approached me and asked me for my help. Like so many
criminal actions, the ultimate resolution of this case involved some
very pragmatic decisions by both the prosecution and defense
teams, compromises both sides accepted. Yet these compromises led
to a resolution of the case that ultimately failed to satisfy any of the
individuals affected by these murders. This is a story of American
justice, but with a Chinese flavor.

THE FACTS OF THE CASE

Tseng Jyi "Jimi" Peng became a very successful Taiwanese businessman whose manufacturing companies produced and marketed
CB radios, electronic speakers, and other electronic products. Lisa
was born in Taiwan city. She was the second of eight siblings. Her

father passed away when she was very young. Her mother raised all eight children. After Lisa graduated from college, she started working at an electronic supplier, TWA. She and Jimi met in 1972 while they both worked for TWA. Soon afterward they fell in love and got married. Twenty years later, the two started their own company, Sunbern. The couple eventually had two children, both of them boys, who went through elementary and secondary schools in Taiwan. For her part, Lisa not only raised her sons, Michael and Alan, and filled the role of the traditional homemaker for her husband and family, but she also served as treasurer of the new company. Much of the original investment capital Jimi used to start his electronics manufacturing business was borrowed from his wife's family and friends. The company got off the ground. With the help of his wife, Peng's corporate successes continued to gather steam during the late eighties as he was able to tap into the global electronics market that was taking shape, and he launched several spin-off companies. Eventually, Jimi consolidated his companies into a single entity, the Ranger Corporation, which was extremely successful. Peng's personal fortune would soon be estimated at $200 million.[1]

As the economic relations between Taiwan and China's government began to normalize, his corporation thrived and Peng began to make plans to diversify into computers and to establish manufacturing facilities on the Chinese mainland for his electronic products. He first built a manufacturing plant in Shanghai and then began to look toward northern China for further expansion, focusing on the Quin Dao City. Because of the demands his business put on him, Jimi often found himself on the road for weeks at a time, a fact that his family in Taiwan had to accept as the price of his success. In August 1990, on one of his frequent trips, Peng met Ranbing "Jennifer" Ji, an attractive twenty-two-year-old hotel public relations receptionist, at an electronics convention. The two soon became romantically involved, and Jimi, during one of his return trips to Quin Dao, asked Jennifer to take a permanent job with his business. Jimi paid her $300 for her expenses. He also gave her two skirts. She gave Jimi a used T-shirt with lipstick on the collar in return. Several months later he asked Jennifer to move to Shanghai to become assistant manager of his office there.

Her salary would be 750 yuan, the equivalent of $100 per month, a large salary by Shanghai standards at the time.

Jimi had also started to look toward the United States and the enormous potential that the American market held for his lines of electronic products. In the early nineties, Jimi established Ranger Communications in San Diego. He bought a home in Rancho Santa Margarita, Orange County, California, near the University of California at Irvine, where his older son had enrolled. Meanwhile, Jennifer Ji was having difficulty putting down roots in Shanghai, and she also discovered that she was pregnant with her boss's baby. In December of 1992, Jimi moved his mistress to the United States and rented an apartment for her in Mission Viejo, a small, middle-class Orange County town, not far from Anaheim. Peng also gave Jennifer Ji money for her to start a new business affiliated with his company. In March of 1993, Jennifer Ji gave birth to the couple's son, giving him an American name, Kevin.

Lisa Peng later said that, prior to August of 1993, she did not know her husband was having an affair in China with another woman. Before that discovery, Mrs. Peng had concentrated on helping Jimi expand their corporation. She had felt that up to that point, the family had lived in harmony. When Mrs. Peng was auditing the family's phone bill in August of 1993, she found a disproportionate number of calls had been made to Jennifer Ji. Subsequently, she found a woman's T-shirt with red lipstick on it. When she confronted her husband, Jimi admitted that the shirt had been given to him by Jennifer Ji. Lisa Peng immediately phoned Jennifer Ji and confronted her about the shirt. Jennifer denied that the shirt had any special meaning and said that it had been given to Jimi Peng in a lighthearted way.

Jimi Peng contradicted this timeline and said that, in late 1992, he had admitted to his wife that he had been romantically involved with Jennifer Ji. Mrs. Peng, who still lived in Taiwan but frequently visited the United States, was at first outwardly calm about this news, according to Peng. She had seemed to accept the fact that her husband was in a relationship with another woman and that he was about to father a child with her. However, according to Jimi Peng, this stoic response soon turned to anger. In February of 1993, using her house key, Lisa Peng had made a surprise visit to the home she and her husband owned in Rancho Santa Margarita, and she discovered Jennifer Ji living there. Finding Ji's clothing in the bedroom closets and strewn about the master bedroom, Mrs. Peng became so furious that she took scissors and cut these garments into pieces. Mrs. Peng later confronted Jennifer Ji, then eight months pregnant, in a phone call and threatened her with bodily harm if Ji did not stay away from her husband.

Lisa Peng soon began to implore her husband to give up his mistress and threatened to divorce him if he persisted in seeing Jennifer Ji. Peng finally acquiesced and went to Ji with an offer of $300,000 for her to get out of his life. Jennifer Ji countered by asking Jimi to divorce Lisa and marry her. She also wanted Jimi Peng to purchase a home for her son and herself, costing an additional $800,000. Peng balked at the $1.1 million amount. On August 15, 1993, Lisa Peng left Taiwan to visit her son in the United States. She had heard about Jennifer Ji's economic demands and, like her husband, thought that the $1.1 million was an absolutely unacceptable and excessive amount. Up to this time, Jimi Peng had stayed with his wife but had continued to visit Jennifer Ji whenever the opportunity presented itself. Later on in court, the defense argued that Jennifer Ji had begun to break away from her status as Jimi Peng's mistress.[2]

THE INVESTIGATION OF THE CASE

On August 18, 1993, Jimi Peng purportedly arrived at Jennifer Ji's apartment at 21622 Marger Erite Parkway in Mission Viejo, California. He had just returned from a trip to Hong Kong. He rang the doorbell, and no one answered. Getting no response at the apartment, Jimi then decided to wait for Jennifer's return in the manager's office of the building, where he stayed until 5:30 PM, when the manager closed the office. Jimi returned to the apartment and again tried the doorbell and got no response. So he left a note on the door. Then he wandered around the complex until 11:00 that evening. He

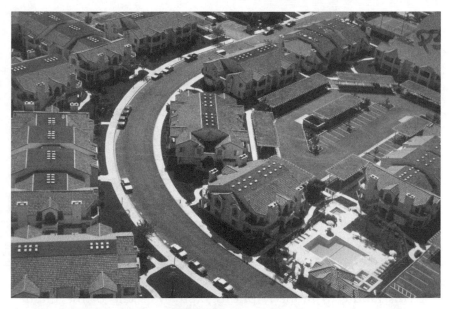

Aerial view of the crime scene and residence.

went back to Ji's apartment and, still getting no response, decided to find a way inside. Jimi's narrative of what happened next and other details in this case are very ably provided in the Chinese-language book *Who Killed Ji Ranbing?* by Qi Sing Wu, published in 1999.[3]

Finding the front door of the apartment unlocked, Jimi later recalled that he let himself in, switched on a light, and discovered Jennifer's bloody body in a slightly upright position on the living-room floor adjacent to a couch. He tried to lift her, but discovered her body was cold. Jennifer was wearing a black dress with white polka dots, and her underpants had been pulled down to her knees. Her right hand was holding a baby's bib, and her left hand was over her chest. Jimi would later testify that he noticed multiple bloody wounds on Jennifer's body and a baby's milk bottle lying on the floor next to her left foot. He did not have a cell phone at this time and was unable to get through on the apartment's telephone. He next went into the bathroom, where he relieved himself. He then went to a neighbor's apartment and called the police. He told the police dispatcher, "My wife has been murdered."

The Mission Viejo police and Orange County sheriff's deputies arrived at the crime scene within minutes of Jimi Peng's call, and they quickly cordoned off the crime scene. Investigators soon established that Jennifer was not Jimi's wife, but his mistress. They quickly assessed the victim's multiple stab wounds and found a green pillow lying on the couch, with one side covered by blood and the other side showing small amounts of blood spatter. Investigators then searched the rest of the apartment, and in the baby's bedroom they found Kevin Ji dead in his crib, with a small piece of baby clothing stuffed in his mouth. Jimi Peng acknowledged that he was the father of his mistress's dead child. A medical responder then removed the cloth from Kevin Ji's mouth and found that it was a portion of the baby's own T-shirt. No photographs were taken to document the position of the dead infant's body or the condition of the T-shirt cloth found in his mouth.

This failure to properly photograph the scene of the infant's murder later proved an important oversight, one that would become crucial in court. It came down to the question: did someone intentionally stuff the shirt into Kevin Ji's mouth, or, during the ordeal, did Kevin become extremely hungry and, while he frantically cried, did he swallow a corner of his own T-shirt, suffocating himself? Establishing either of these two contrasting scenarios could determine whether a court found his death a homicide or an accidental death. In the subsequent autopsy, the coroner, Dr. Joseph J. Halka, found that Jennifer Ji had been stabbed nineteen times with a single-bladed knife, in all likelihood a kitchen knife. There was a wound to the victim's right cheek, shallow and five inches long, and a second stab wound to the upper-left chest, one and a half inches deep. One possible fatal wound was also to the left chest, only lower, and it pierced Ji's left lung. There were three more stab wounds to the left chest, two of them surface and a third that penetrated the aorta, causing massive bleeding, another fatal wound. Three of the wounds were to the victim's left arm, most likely defensive in nature, and to her left wrist and ring finger. Another wound indicated that the victim turned her back to her assailant. The pattern of wounds indicated that Jennifer had put up a brief and spirited fight, but the collective nature of the wounds quickly rendered her defenseless. Police found a bloodlike substance on the inside of the apartment's door and on the outside hallway, immediately next to the door. Yet investigators found no blood trail leading from the couch to the front door.

Police investigators quickly focused on Jimi Peng as their principal suspect, questioning him for several hours. Subsequent DNA testing confirmed that he was, in fact, Kevin's father. There was no evidence of a forced entry, so the victim, in all probability, knew her assailant. Jimi had a strong motive for wanting Jennifer Ji and their infant son out of his life. And Peng had no plausible alibi for the time of death, established at midmorning to midday of August 18, except for the period of time he had spent in the building manager's office. Detectives found a single brass garment button on the carpeted floor of the living room, one that could be worn on either a man's or a woman's clothing. However, the police had discovered a bite mark on the victim's left arm, and the bite mark did not match Jimi Peng's teeth. Also, there were no bloodstains found on his clothing, and, moreover, police, aware that Jennifer Ji had put up a spirited defense, did not find any injuries to his body. Jimi also passed a polygraph test. Subsequently, the police eliminated Jimi Peng as a suspect.[4]

What happened in the next few months would ultimately prove to be a nightmare for the authorities, as they switched the focus of their investigation from Jimi Peng to his wife, Lisa Peng. Jimi Peng offered to help the Orange County sheriff's deputies investigating the case by taking them to his home in Santa Marguerita to show them his wife's clothing and her financial records. Peng himself searched his wife's clothing, looking for a missing brass button. On August 25, investigating deputies found Jennifer's damaged clothing left in Lisa Peng's closets. In the coming weeks, Peng offered a large reward for anyone helping to convict those responsible for the murders. During this time span, Mrs. Peng returned to Taiwan, which had no extradition treaty with the United States.

In January of 1994, in a critical move, Peng convinced his wife that she should return to the United States to assist police investiga-

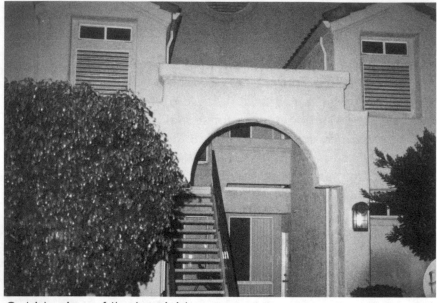

Outside view of the homicide scene.

tors. As soon as Lisa arrived in Los Angeles, deputies quickly brought her to the county lockup. There they grilled her on the murders for four hours, without giving her a *Miranda* warning: that she had the right to remain silent and the right to an attorney and that anything she said could be used against her in a court of law. This questioning took place in a basement room at the jail. Mrs. Peng repeatedly asked for a lawyer, a request that the investigators did not honor. At this juncture, Jimi Peng offered to act as an interpreter for the investigators, using their native Taiwanese dialect for the remainder of a nine-hour interview.

The deputies, without Mrs. Peng's knowledge, secretly wired Jimi and taped all of this grilling. As he took his wife aside to talk to her quietly, Mr. Peng, knowing that the conversation was being recorded, drew out from his wife an admission that she had gone to Jennifer's apartment earlier on the day of the murder and had confronted her in a very angry manner. Lisa admitted that she had demanded that Jennifer get out of her husband's life and take her son with her. Then, thinking only her husband would hear what she had to say, Lisa Peng broke into tears and admitted that she had bitten Jennifer on her left arm during this heated conversation. Sheriff's investigators continued to interview Lisa Peng. For about nine hours in total she was at no time afforded access to a lawyer. Advised by Jimi Peng that his wife had admitted visiting Jennifer Ji on August 18 and that she had bitten Jennifer, the sheriff's office arrested Lisa Peng for the double murder. Lisa was immediately confined to prison since the courts recognized that this defendant posed a serious threat of fleeing to Taiwan. Subsequently, the Orange County crime lab tested Lisa Peng's DNA and found that it matched the DNA in the saliva taken from the bite mark on Jennifer's left arm. At Lisa's preliminary hearing, Jimi Peng testified that his wife had told him she would give up their marriage if he really loved Jennifer and wanted to marry her.

Lisa Peng's 1994 arrest for these murders created a media sensation in not only the Chinese community in the United States but also in Taiwan and throughout Asia. Her picture and lurid accounts of how Jennifer and Kevin had been savagely murdered were featured on the front page of all the major Chinese papers. In contrast to this, the case received little attention from the California press and the local TV newscasts.[5]

I had first heard about these murders in later August of 1993 when I received a phone call from Margaret Kuo, a good friend and colleague of mine who was the assistant director of the Orange County Sheriff's Department Forensic Laboratory. Kuo was assisting in investigating the Ji murders. Margaret Kuo and I had worked together on several projects over a period of twenty years or so. She is a very capable and respected forensic scientist, and we had developed a solid professional relationship. We talked by telephone in our native Chinese a couple of times a year, discussing various issues facing the forensic community. We also bumped into one another at national symposiums and forensic conferences about twice a year. Sitting in my office at the Connecticut State Police Forensic Science Laboratory in Meriden, I listened as Margaret provided me with the particulars on the case against Lisa Peng. Since I had plans to attend an annual symposium at the FBI lab in a few weeks, I suggested to

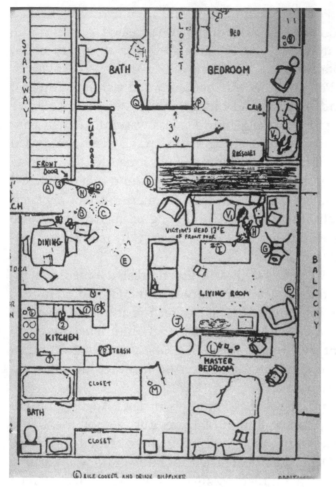

Crime scene
diagram.

Margaret that she should bring the crime scene photos and documents to show me when we got to the FBI academy in Quantico, Virginia, as she later did.

I studied the dozen photos that Margaret provided me, and I tentatively reached the following conclusions:

- The scene is a typical indoor, primary crime scene. Jennifer was killed in the living room.
- There was no forced entry; the victim could have known the assailant or assailants.

- Jennifer died of multiple knife wounds. The homicide weapon was most likely a kitchen knife.
- More likely than not, this crime was committed by more than one assailant.
- This crime had all the earmarks of a crime of passion.
- Kevin's death could have been an accident but was not necessarily an accident.

Finally, the lack of a blood trail from the victim's couch to her apartment door, where more blood was discovered, particularly interested me. I advised her that there could have been more than one assailant and that the case bore the earmarks of a crime of passion. Other than those observations, I do not recall any other critical insights from that viewing of the dozen crime scene photos. I did suggest that if the detectives needed any help, they could contact me directly. In 1994 I chaired an international forensic conference in Taiwan, where Margaret Kuo made an excellent presentation on the Lisa Peng case. Her presentation was basically about the scientific fact that the DNA

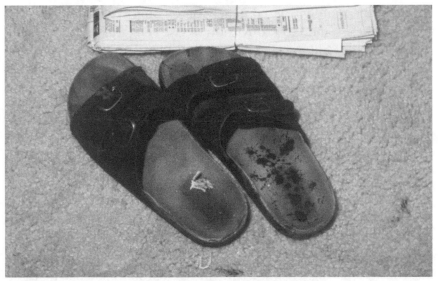

A pair of sandals were found near the doorway. Low-velocity vertical blood droplets were found on only the right sandal. Nothing was found on the left one.

taken from the bite mark established Lisa Peng as its source without commenting on any other specific facts of the crime.

Lisa Peng was prosecuted for the double murders in Orange County in late 1994. Members of Jennifer Ji's family traveled from China to attend the trial. This proceeding led to a mistrial being declared in early 1995 with the jury deadlocked, ten for a conviction and two for acquittal. Prosecutors moved ahead with a second trial, also attended by the Ji family, and in a Santa Ana courtroom on April 25, 1996, Lisa Peng was convicted of the second-degree murder of Jennifer Ji and the first-degree murder of Kevin, her infant son. Ms. Peng was then sentenced to life in prison without parole and was incarcerated in the California State Penitentiary at Chino. All of these developments continued to generate great interest in the California Chinese American community and in the Chinese-language media. The case was also heavily covered by the media in Taiwan and China. This set off numerous demonstrations due to the issues inherent in the trial, such as the family tragedies the case caused, as well as the critical fact of a successful Chinese businessman having a second, "secret wife."[6] Eventually, a movie was made on the murders, based largely on Qi Sing Wu's book.

Nonetheless, the 1996 conviction of Lisa Peng was overturned by a 3–0 vote by the California Fourth District Court of Appeals in Santa Ana on October 4, 1999. This decision was based on the interrogation tactics used by investigators during the nine-hour grilling given to Lisa Peng in a basement office of the jail in January of 1994, without her being advised of her *Miranda* rights. The judges also condemned the sheriffs' investigators for using her husband, Jimi Peng, as both an interpreter and as an interrogator. Finally, the court also criticized the investigators for secretly taping Lisa during her nine-hour ordeal. After reviewing their situation, the Orange County prosecutors office decided to appeal the lower court's decision to the California Supreme Court, which on January 19, 2000, upheld the court of appeals reversal of the conviction. Lisa Peng remained in prison during these legal proceedings, since she was considered a flight risk and since the United States still had no extradition treaty with Taiwan. On January 24, Orange County prosecutors announced that they would seek a third trial of Mrs. Peng.

During my visits to Taiwan, Mrs. Peng's friends made contact with me to ask me to assist Lisa Peng in fighting what they perceived as a profound injustice. She had, from the very time of the double murder, maintained her innocence, and her children and other family members in Taiwan believed her. They believed, instead, that Lisa's husband, Jimi Peng, had committed the two murders. I could not ignore the family's terrible suffering, nor could I forget the strange nature of the crime scene photos that I had viewed. As I remembered those images, it seemed inconceivable to me that a small, middle-aged woman could have perpetrated the savage, multiple stab wounds to Jennifer Ji, let alone follow that up by suffocating an infant. I agreed to take another look at this case. John Barnett, a prominent Los Angeles defense attorney, contacted me in March of 2000. Subsequently, Christopher J. Plourd, a prominent San Diego lawyer with special expertise and extensive knowledge of DNA evidence, contacted Barnett and me. He asked me to serve as the defense's forensic expert when the case came up for retrial. Plourd had also served on several national DNA committees with me. The two of us usually met in Washington, DC, and in Chicago to attend meetings, and afterward we talked late into the night, discussing the scientific merits of the case and investigating the procedures used. When word of my decision reached the prosecution, there was an initial objection over my involvement, since the investigators who had initially contacted me had shown me the crime scene photos. However, the extent of my activity had been deemed "cursory," in Margaret Kuo's words, and the prosecution decided that there would be no point in challenging, as a conflict of interest, my role as part or Mrs. Peng's defense team.

In April of 2000, I flew to California to go over all of the case files and to study very closely all of the crime scene photos and to reexamine all the physical evidence collected by the police. It is always nice to work with truly professional forensic scientists. As I always say, forensic scientists should maintain their independence and objectivity. We are not working for the prosecution or for the defense. The goal of forensic science is to find the scientific facts and the truth. The Orange County Sheriff's Department Forensic Laboratory was, indeed, staffed by consummate professionals. These individuals cooperated with us in every way, and Margaret Kuo's assistants made my reexamination a very smooth and professional process.

Christopher Plourd arrived with me at the laboratory on a sunny Saturday morning. We initiated our examination at about 8:00 AM. We were finished with our examination about 6:00 PM. We examined a total of twenty-five items of forensic evidence. These are our most important findings:

- A large, bloody handprint was noted on the reverse side of the green pillow that was found on the sofa next to Jennifer's body. Although there were no usable finger or palm print details that could be taken from this handprint, it was noted that the hand was sufficiently larger than a small woman's hand.
- A whole apple peel was found in the garbage can in the kitchen. This apple peel was peeled in a perfect fashion, from the top to the bottom as a whole, and with no breaks in it. No apple traces were found in Jennifer's stomach contents. Who peeled and ate this apple? We later discovered that Jimi Peng habitually peeled apples in this manner.
- No fingerprints, shoe prints, bloodstains, or other physical evidence was found at the crime scene that could be linked to Lisa Peng.
- Lisa was in her fifties and was very slender and small, while Jennifer was in her midtwenties and was very strong and athletic. She was decades younger than Lisa. It was almost impossible for such a violent attack to occur without Lisa sustaining any physical injuries.
- A metal button was found at the crime scene. This button clearly was there as a result of a struggle. It was established that this button did not emanate from any clothing worn or owned by either Lisa or Jennifer. It could have come from clothing worn by the assailant.
- This crime scene is obviously a primary crime scene, without any sign of breaking and entering. Jennifer was overpowered and stabbed nineteen times. Was this crime really committed

by one person? Or were there one or more additional individuals involved?

The third trial of Lisa Peng started in April of 2001, before California Superior Court Judge William R. Froeberg. For the third time,
Jennifer Ji's parents and other family members flew in from China
to attend the trial. Lisa Peng's sons also attended. Since the earlier
jury had not found Mrs. Peng guilty of first-degree murder, because
of the doctrine of double jeopardy (a defendant cannot ever be
retried for a crime once a jury has returned a not guilty verdict on a
specific count), the prosecution was forced to put Ms. Peng on trial
for the second-degree murder of Jennifer Ji and made the same
charge for the son's murder. Still, the special circumstance of a multiple murder would prevail, and the prosecutors could demand,
upon both convictions, that Lisa Peng be sentenced to jail for the
rest of her life, without any chance of parole. John Barnett called me
to testify for the defense in mid-May. During my testimony, one
point I emphasized was the absence of any bloody clothing worn by
the assailant ever being found. The only bloody clothing found was
what Jennifer Ji had been wearing. The nature of the nineteen stab
wounds would surely have led to a substantial amount of blood
spatter, much of which would surely have been deposited on the
clothing and person of Jennifer Ji's attacker. Under questioning from
John Barnett, I also noted that Jimi Peng had arrived from Taiwan
early on the morning of August 18, and one witness testified that he
had been carrying three suitcases. Jimi later told investigators he had
only two suitcases. I suggested that the dispensing of the third suitcase could provide a key to solving this case. During the trial, the
prosecution could not use any of the evidence developed in 1994
during the nine hours of interrogation that took place without a
lawyer being present. Also, prosecutors could not introduce any evidence of Lisa Peng's telling her husband that she had visited Jennifer
a day before her murder and had bitten her on the left arm. The
freshness of the bite mark also became a critical issue in the trial. To
preserve the bite-mark evidence, the medical examiner had surgi-
cally removed the flesh on the victim's left arm from around the

wound and the flesh containing the bite mark itself and had this all frozen. This procedure eliminated the possibility of using the original intact arm flesh as evidence of when the bite had actually occurred. Barnett then introduced evidence that the bite, which came from Lisa Peng because it matched her teeth, had not been inflicted at the time of the murder. Instead, Barnett argued that Lisa Peng, was, in fact, a visitor to Jennifer Ji's apartment eighteen hours before her death.[7] The discovery of the apple peel and bloody handprint on the pillow by defense experts also became a bombshell for the prosecution's case. The prosecution had to ask for a recess to consult forensic experts from the Orange County crime lab to prepare to cross-examine me about those issues.

The prosecution gave its closing arguments before the jury of eight men and four women on June 4, 2001. In their summation, the prosecution argued that while Lisa Peng had been very badly wronged by her husband and Jennifer, this did not give Lisa the right to kill her husband's lover and the infant boy whom the couple's relationship had produced. The jury could even feel sympathy for the defendant, yet convict her of these crimes. In his defense summation, John Barnett argued that Jimi Peng had committed the murders and that the crimes were just about cash, $1.1 million. Under California law, the defense cannot argue that another person committed a murder, unless there is evidence to support this theory. Barnett pointed out that Jimi's behaviors at the crime scene and his statements constituted this evidence, and Judge Froeberg agreed. Instead of Mrs. Peng being the killer, Barnett argued that Jimi Peng was the murderer. His motive was clear, according to Barnett. Lisa Peng "was not being held up for ransom like Jimi Peng was," Barnett declared. Jennifer Ji and Peng had already broken up, he charged, and, prior to her murder, she was beginning to express an interest in finding another career or another man. The case went to the jury on Tuesday, June 5, 2001. On June 18, the jury told Judge Froeberg that they were hopelessly deadlocked, eight for conviction and four for acquittal. The judge then declared a mistrial and set June 29 as the date for the hearing on whether the case would go to trial for a fourth time.

A surprising announcement was made on Friday, June 29, 2001. Orange County prosecutors agreed to allow Lisa Peng to plead guilty to two counts of voluntary manslaughter and one count of the illegal use of a weapon, the knife used to stab Jennifer Ji nineteen times. As part of this compromise, Lisa was sentenced by Judge Froeberg to eleven years for five-month-old Kevin's death and six years for Jennifer's death, sentences that were to run concurrently. However, Lisa received credit for the nearly seven and a half years she had already been imprisoned and could be immediately deported. She was turned over to the United State Immigration and Naturalization Service. In accepting these pleas, Judge Froeberg said, "The court is satisfied that the factual basis for voluntary manslaughter has been proven." The prosecution pointed to the three prior trials as a basis for their entering into this compromise. Jennifer's sister expressed her dissatisfaction with the jury system of this country.[8]

Defense attorney John Barnett called this outcome "not a perfect solution." He added that "if you have an option of going home . . . or waiting six more months in custody (an overestimate of the time required for the deportation proceedings), you go home. . . . Given the options she [Lisa Peng] chose the only viable option." Thus, Lisa Peng would be released in the next month when the deportation process was completed, instead of having to serve the final three and a half years of her sentence. When Lisa Peng arrived in Taiwan in later July, the authorities there questioned her about the two murders. With all the publicity that the murders of Jennifer and Kevin Ji had generated, Ms. Peng was a marked woman when she set foot in Taipei. Under Taiwanese law, a citizen convicted of crimes in another country can, upon returning home, be prosecuted for these same crimes. But Lisa Peng's long ordeal was drawing to a close. Lisa denied committing the two crimes and told investigators that she had been forced to plead guilty to the lesser charges of manslaughter only to gain her freedom and return home. The Taiwanese authorities, I am happy to say, agreed that there was insufficient evidence to prove that Lisa, in fact, was the individual who murdered the two victims, and they chose not to prosecute Lisa Peng. Today she lives in Taiwan as a free woman.

THE SUMMARY

In the quote that began this chapter, I spoke about the vital importance in telling the truth and not trying to paper over the problems in the justice system. Who can really be happy with the outcome of the Lisa Peng case? Certainly not Jennifer's family. Lisa was never found guilty of murder in the first degree in a trial that stood the test of a legal review. Her punishment, accordingly, did not begin to match the terrible loss Jennifer's family must have endured. And, of course, Lisa could not have been happy at feeling herself coerced into confessing to two crimes that she denies ever committing.

If Lisa Peng did not stab Jennifer to death and then suffocate little Kevin, then who did? Who really knows? There was no forcible entry into the victim's apartment, so Jennifer must have known the assailant or assailants. Indeed, given earlier confrontations with Lisa, the victim would, in all likelihood, not have allowed her lover's wife into her home. Jimi, on the other hand, had visited there often. More important, Jimi had a motive for wanting his lover out of his life. Even for someone with a net worth of $200 million, Jennifer's demand for $1.1 million must have represented a staggering blow. Because Jimi had passed a polygraph test (as did Richard Crafts, the woodchipper killer) and was willing to cooperate with the authorities, the Orange County sheriff's office shifted their focus to Lisa Peng as their one and only suspect. Tunnel vision of this sort has caused problems with many investigations in the past. And let us think, for a moment, about the terrible nature of these crimes. Would a slender woman in her early fifties have the strength and sustained power to stab a much younger and more athletic victim nineteen times? Couldn't a much younger victim evade, for at least a time, such an attack? Then, could any normal person approach the crib of a sleeping infant and smother this baby to death? Could a third person, perhaps a hired assassin, murder both Jennifer and Kevin? If the hired assassin is a plausible theory, then who was behind all of this?

So why did Lisa Peng ever plead guilty to the voluntary manslaughter charges? She had been in jail for crimes she had not committed for almost seven and a half years. Her two sons had grown into manhood while she was in jail. Naturally enough, Lisa Peng wanted her life back, what was left of it. If you consider her experiences in this country, is it any wonder that she yearned to return to her homeland and to resume her life there as best she could? Jennifer Ji's sister was right. There are terrible problems with the jury system as it is applied in this country. But it is still the best system ever devised to protect the rights of the innocent while punishing the guilty.

Here, please allow me to add a nota bene. In the past few decades, a new and destructive social phenomenon has occurred. Married and successful Taiwanese businessmen have been going to China to expand their corporations. Over there, they often meet a much younger, beautiful, and aggressive woman, tempting them to forget their oaths to their wives and families. These new relationships often go forward into a full-fledged affair, meaning the new couple lives together. This phenomenon is now referred to as "having a second wife." Many types of family tragedies result from this social phenomenon. The Chinese government has passed a law to prohibit this type of temporary and unofficial extramarital arrangement. Scholars have held symposia and workshops to address this growing social problem. In the case of Jennifer's and Kevin's deaths, the tragedy is all too apparent. Lisa and Jimi Peng's family breakdown is just another example of the kind of tragedy that this social phenomenon can cause.

Nevertheless, the law, the jury system, trials, and forensic science will not be able to resolve these social issues. Every day we see new cases identical to what befell Jennifer, Kevin, Lisa, and Jimi. As a matter of fact, there are hundreds, even thousands, of Jennifers, Kevins, Lisas, and Jimis whose tragedies are waiting to happen in Taiwan, Hong Kong, China, the United States, and elsewhere around the world. Unless, of course, we, as husbands and fathers, learn to control our desires and temptations. And unless the women who are tempted to take on a wealthy businessman learn to respect other women's rights, their families, and their own lives. Unless this happens, history will repeat itself. I hope that this case serves as a wake-up call for not only the Chinese community, but also for our entire global society.

As I told the University of New Haven graduates on that commencement day, the world is full of pitfalls and injustices. We, as citizens, simply have to do our best to right the wrongs and to move forward to a better world for our children and their children.

CHAPTER FIVE

THE SUZAN BARRATT CASE

BLOOD WILL TELL THE TALE

The faster you want to fulfill your destiny,
the slower you will get there.

—Ancient Chinese proverb

F orensic investigators have very interesting jobs, but this work often requires long, tedious, and painstaking work. The hours that a dedicated forensic investigator must put in to meet the complex demands that routine assignments place on him require a willingness to spend days, weekends, and even weeks away from family and friends. On call seven days a week, the forensic investigator must provide timely service, since much forensic evidence is, by definition, perishable. Thus, the earlier that physical evidence can be found, collected, and properly examined, the better the chances are that a case can be successfully solved. So it is not at all uncommon for the forensic scientist to be called away from formal family gatherings, including holidays. Add to this the constant court appearances and special training required to perform these duties, and one can easily see why there is a high burnout rate in forensic investigative work. And all the while, the forensic professional must keep current on the latest scientific breakthroughs in the discipline, as well as the evolving legal precedents that affect the investigator's daily work.

Forensic scientists are trained to use their analytical abilities, relying heavily on applied logic. It is absolutely essential for the investigator to keep an open mind. Meanwhile, police detectives and investigators are also trained to use their own instincts and powers of observation, while withholding judgement. However, even very experienced forensic scientists and police detectives can jump to a conclusion without considering a range of appropriate scientific and logical hypotheses. This is regrettable but very true. It is at times very difficult for veteran investigators to remain objective about each crime they investigate. There is, for instance, the constant temptation to look at a specific set of facts through the prism of past experience. If a crime was committed six months ago and today's call to a crime scene immediately seems to present a picture that closely resembles that of a half year earlier, then there is a natural inclination for the investigator to start jumping to conclusions. Premature conclusions. Conclusions that prompt the unwary investigator to take steps that later analyses prove unwise. Once taken, investigators can have a very difficult time in changing their minds and the direction of an investigation, or even the prosecution of a particular suspect. This problem can be compounded many times over by the media. Pressures from superiors and from the families of the victims only add to what can become a rush to judgment. The police want to perform expeditiously and well, and they want to have that excellent performance publicly recognized. Put another way, like all other public agencies, police departments do not like to step backward and admit to a mistake.

By their very nature, terrible crimes committed within a community provoke wide and immediate public alarm and interest. The media are only responding to the public's right to know when they swarm to the scene of some horrific event or what appears on its face value to be a high-profile case, such as a homicide. The pressure mounts to find the culprit—and quickly. And the rush to judgment can result in a mistake. None of the professionals I have known over the years, police or otherwise, like to admit they've made a mistake. This is simply human nature, or so it seems to me.

The Suzan Barratt case presents a graphic example of how competent and very experienced forensic investigators can quickly draw erroneous conclusions from the scene of a premature death, one that appears to them to represent a homicide. A fact that investigators keep in mind when responding to a domestic call is that 70 to 80 percent of all homicides are committed by an individual who knows the victim. If the chronic abuse of alcohol is a factor in the domestic call, the responding investigators can be even more inclined to view matters in a formulaic fashion. The Barratt case is important in showing how the total canvas has to be closely and professionally studied before setting an investigation on a specific course, one designed to realize a specific legal outcome.

THE FACTS OF THE CASE

Stephen Haines, forty-six, lived with his fiancée, Suzan Barratt, also forty-six, in a home they rented in Port St. Lucie, Florida, part of that state's famed Treasure Coast region. The overall area is one of the most beautiful in the country, featuring miles of beachfront leading down to the glistening waters of the Atlantic Ocean. During the winter months, thousands of people from the North, sometimes referred to as snowbirds, bask in its plentiful sunshine. Tourists stay there in February and March to watch major league baseball teams, such as the New York Mets, go through their annual spring training process. Port St. Lucie itself is a small community. Many of its residents are retirees from up north or individuals from other parts of the country, like Haines and Barratt, who moved there to start a new life. By October of 1999, this couple had been together for eighteen months. Stephen Haines had lived in the Port St. Lucie area since

1981 and had for years owned a concession stand on the beach. He then closed it down and took a job as an auto mechanic at Coastal Car Care in Stuart, Florida. Suzan Barratt, who was a real estate agent, originally came from New Jersey and moved to Florida with her mother following her father's death. Haines was a known alcoholic, and Barratt was also a heavy drinker. (During the latter portion of this investigation, she would be arrested for driving under the influence of alcohol.) The couple's friends and neighbors were well aware of their heavy-drinking habits. Elaine Barratt, Suzan's mother, did not like Stephen Haines and had told her daughter's boyfriend on Mother's Day of 1998 that he was not welcome in her home on nearby Hutchinson Island.

On Monday, October 4, 1999, police received a late-morning 911 call from Elaine Barratt, Suzan's mother, who said her distraught daughter had reported finding Haines's naked, dead body lying on the floor of their home's garage at about 11:00 AM. The Port St. Lucie police responded to the scene, and detectives soon arrived. They found Stephen Haines's body facedown on the floor of the garage, with a small amount of blood serum running from his face to the north wall. A large number of bruises and abrasion marks could be seen covering his body. Bloodstains and blood smearings were all over the garage floor. A washer and dryer were observed in the corner adjacent to the door leading into the house. Detectives found several shirts, pants, and towels, heavily stained with blood, inside the washer. These articles were immediately seized as evidence. The investigators followed a trail of blood drops into a small hallway that led to the kitchen. In the kitchen, large amounts of blood drops and blood smears were found. The living room was adjacent to the kitchen. In it detectives found bloody footprints on the floor. In the living room they moreover discovered two bloodstains on the floor that resembled the shape of a human body. Additional blood drops were also discovered around the living room. Detectives furthermore found a few fragments of green-colored broken glass on the floor, amid the bloodstains. Following the blood drops, detectives found more blood smears and blood spatters on the bathroom floor. They also saw a reddish liquid and bloodlike matter in the toilet bowl. Additionally, the detectives saw signs of someone having washed and cleaned up the tub, which still had blood residue. In this detailed search, the investigators also found more bloodstains throughout the house and a washed rug hanging on the picnic table in the backyard, with a reddish, bloodlike liquid still dripping from it onto the cement patio floor under the picnic table.

After the medical examiner arrived at the scene, Stephen Haines's body was turned over. Upon examination, police investigators saw more bruises and blood smears on his body. In addition, a laceration was found on the area around the bridge of his nose. This laceration appeared to have resulted from a cut with a sharp instrument. Since broken glass fragments were found on the living-room floor, a major effort was launched to look for a homicide weapon. Searching through the garbage can, investigators found an empty wine bottle that had what appeared to be brownish traces on it. On the curb in front of the house, they found a white garbage bag that contained scores of empty beer cans, bottles, and bloody

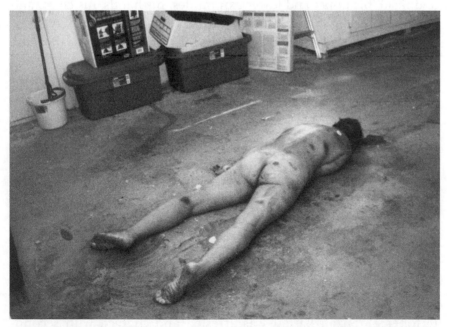

Stephen Haines's body was found on the garage floor of his house.

tissues. Suzan Barratt, who had spent the previous night at home, was sitting in a living-room chair when police arrived and seemed to be most intent on cleaning up her residence. She complained loudly about all of the blood and persistently asked the investigators to leave her house. Police noticed that Barratt's right forearm was swollen, and that there were fresh scraping marks on her knuckles. Investigators also observed dried blood under her fingernails and small amounts of dried blood on her feet and legs. During questioning, Barratt told investigators that Haines suffered from a chronic alcohol-induced blood condition that caused him to bleed profusely whenever he received a skin laceration. The investigators noted that Barratt did not seem to show any grief over her fiancé's death during this initial interview.

Dr. Frederick Hobin, the St. Lucie County's medical examiner, performed an autopsy on Haines the evening of October 4. He found that Haines had died of "multiple contusion [deep bruise] injuries." He reported finding 140 injury marks over Haines's face and head, his upper and lower extremities, his hands, his chest, and his back, as well as three broken ribs. Based on his own observations and the police investigative reports, Dr. Hobin ruled that the manner of death was a homicide and that Haines had been beaten to death by blunt objects. Earlier on October 4, police questioned Suzan Barratt for four hours at the Port St. Lucie police station without providing her with any *Miranda* warning, even after she had inquired about the possibility of obtaining the services of a lawyer. During this prolonged interview, investigators were able to extract additional information from Barratt. She finally told police that Haines and she had argued loudly the night before his body was discovered and that she had struck her fiancé several times, kicking him, and hitting him once with a wine bottle. Barratt said that, following this altercation, she had fled into the bedroom, while Haines went into the bathroom. Around midnight, when Barratt came out of the bedroom, she saw Haines drinking a beer.

On October 6 police ruled Haines's death a homicide, and on October 15 Suzan Barratt was arrested and charged with second-degree manslaughter. Barratt was initially held in the Port St. Lucie

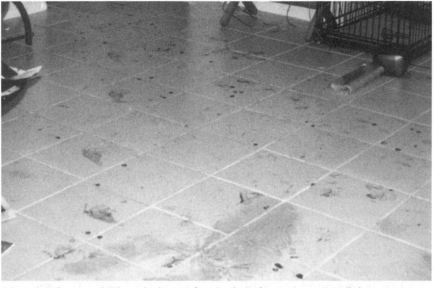

Bloodstains and bloody bare footprints found on the living-room floor.

County jail without bail. Within a few days, Barratt had retained defense attorney Richard D. Kibbey of Stuart, Florida, to represent her. Kibbey asked for and was granted a bail-bond hearing, and Barratt was released, pending trial, after posting $100,000 bail.

Richard Kibbey, a seasoned and bright lawyer, has been in practice in that area for many years and has earned an excellent reputation. He studied the crime scene photos, and, to his experienced eye, the blood evidence did not seem to bear out the police contention that Stephen Haines had left the substantial blood spattering inside his home as a result of being beaten to death. Kibbey saw blood smears, such as might be left behind by someone struggling to move from room to room. In November of 1999, Valerie Shook, my very able assistant at the Connecticut State Police Forensic Laboratory in Meriden, began to receive phone calls from Richard Kibbey, asking to speak with me about the case. As usual, I was extremely busy, especially so at that time of year, due to most courts trying to clear their dockets by year's end. As a result, like tax accountants just prior to April 15, lawyers from everywhere seemed to want to call me to testify about their cases before the holiday season. Thus, I wasn't able to return his calls.

However, I was working in my office on November 22, my birthday, when the persistent Mr. Kibbey called me again, and I spoke to him. Listening to his concerns and observations, I realized at once that he was a very genuine and concerned professional. He then convinced me that there were issues of injustice involved in this case. I finally agreed to look over the crime scene photographic evidence and reports he would send me. Two days later, I received Richard Kibbey's huge package, which consisted of the autopsy report, crime scene investigation notes, a synopsis of the statements taken, and over a hundred crime scene photos. Although many of the photos were repetitive in nature, these photos graphically showed that there were large quantities of bloodstains in virtually every room in the house. (One was a photograph of Haines's bloody feet that is presented in the photo insert of this book.) These bloodstains were mainly low-velocity vertical drops, blood smears, and bloody bare footprints. I saw that Richard Kibbey was indeed correct and that the blood evidence that I observed did not appear to be the result of a murder.

There were two observations I made that seemed inconsistent with the injuries described in the autopsy report. First, the amount of blood found throughout the house was inconsistent with Haines's injuries. It is true that, scientifically, we cannot determine the exact amount of blood from photographs. However, with experience, a forensic scientist can estimate and distinguish a small amount of blood from a medium volume or a large amount or an extremely large volume of blood. From the volume of blood and its respective patterns, we can determine the more likely type of injury a person has sustained. For example, if a small cut of soft tissue is visible, only a few drops of blood or a small amount of blood smears would be found at the scene. A more serious cut would produce a greater volume of blood, thus causing multiple deposits. With a cut damaging a vein, the blood usually runs out with a large amount of deposits. Meanwhile, if a cut involved an artery, blood will gush out and will leave a pattern typical of an artery gushing, which resembles multiple blood spatters that look as though they have been shot out of a lawn sprinkler. By studying the scene, the forensic investigator can also distinguish the differences of the bloodstain patterns that result from a simple stab wound versus multiple stab wounds, as well as the loss of a finger versus the loss of a limb, such as an arm or leg. He can also discern the blood patterns of a superficial cut versus a cut throat. The large amount of blood in Haines's residence flatly contradicted a single small cut on his nose as the source. Nor could it be from the 140 multiple contusion-type injuries. Those bloodstains had to come from another source.

Second, the bloodstain patterns found in Haines's house also spelled out a different story than a homicide. Most of the bloodstains found inside the house were blood smears and low-velocity, passive blood drops. Blood smears generally are caused by a small amount of liquid blood transfer from a source to another surface after contact. Low-velocity, passive blood drops are the result of liquid blood dripping out of a source, such as a cut on the nose or vomit out of the mouth, without any additional external or internal forces. At a homicide scene involving severe lacerations or multiple cuts or stab wounds, the forensic investigator usually expects to see different types of bloodstain patterns, such as cast-off blood spatters on the walls or ceiling, artery gushing or spray patterns, and an accumulation of blood pools.

Moreover, the blood drops found on the floor in Haines's home also had a strange pattern, with a hollow/ghost center. I made my initial crime scene observations known to attorney Richard Kibbey and asked him for any additional photographs or videotapes of the scene that he could show me. I was especially interested in close-up views of the blood drops, so I could conduct a more detailed, microscopic study of those blood drops.

At this time I had been very preoccupied with a multiple-agency task force investigation of a serial killer, so it was a few days before I was able to phone Kibbey back. He was delighted to hear from me, especially when I said that I also had problems with calling the blood patterns evidence of a homicide caused by a wine bottle. But

I told Kibbey what I tell all lawyers, whether defense lawyers or prosecutors: I would go only where the physical evidence took me, and nowhere else, whether or not that helped or hurt a particular case. Kibbey quickly agreed to my ground rules. I also told him that the cause of death in this case was certainly the major issue and that he should contact Dr. Joseph Davis, the former Miami-Dade County chief medical examiner, a former president of the American Association of Forensic Scientists and a world-renowned forensic pathologist. Dr. Davis and I had worked on several cases together before. He is more than a world-class forensic pathologist. He is a man with a wall full of testimonials and a person who possesses a great grasp of forensic knowledge. While Mr. Kibbey was enlisting the assistance of Dr. Davis, he also went before the courts and succeeded in having Suzan Barratt declared "partially indigent," so that the state would pay the expenses needed to retain outside experts.

During January of 2000 I was scheduled to give a lecture to a law enforcement conference in south Florida. Good friends of ours, Dr. Frank Chuang and his wife, Lily, invited Margaret and me to stay for a few days in their home in Boca Raton to teach us how to play golf. I told Richard Kibbey that the two of us could meet at a nearby club house and go over the case in detail. Early one afternoon, Kibbey, whom I had never met in person before, arrived, and we quickly found the right chemistry for working together and decided to go downstairs to the club's vacant card room, where we spread out all of the case's reports, documentation, and crime scene photos. We pored over all of this material, some of which I was seeing for the first time. While we were hard at work there, several ladies from the local bridge club began to arrive for their afternoon games. Needless to say, some of these elderly ladies were shocked at the scene that greeted them. Others became very interested in the case and wanted to help. I was gratified that I had a good lawyer present to explain why gruesome photos of a naked dead man adorned their bridge tables. The startled ladies retreated for a few moments to allow us to collect our materials and to make our way to another room, where we continued our intense study and discussion of the evidence. The further I went into this case, the more I appreciated the friendship and support Margaret and I received from Richard Kibbey, his lovely wife, Dana, and his highly efficient and talented administrative assistant, Kelli Wilson. What could have proven an exhaustive trip for Margaret and me to learn to hit the little white golf ball proved to be a stimulating and productive stay to crack another case. Following our conference, Richard and I continued to confer by phone on the blood evidence, more discovery materials, a regional crime laboratory's reports, and additional photographs that had been sent to me. Once back at home, the little laboratory in my house was piled high with material and evidence from the Barratt case. We were then preparing the case for the next legal step, a preliminary hearing that would determine if there was enough evidence to take this case to trial.

On March 22, 2000, Dr. Davis and Kibbey flew to Connecticut to hold a strategy meeting with me in my office at the University of New Haven. The three of us met and reviewed all of the evidence. To accomplish this, we broke down our areas of responsibility according to our expertise: Dr. Joe Davis, the autopsy report and other medical evidence; Richard Kibbey, the investigative reports; and myself, the forensic evidence and crime scene reconstruction. Pressed for time, we worked through lunch, and then I drove the others to Tweed–New Haven Airport for a late-afternoon flight. We discovered that the outgoing flight was delayed, so the three of us found a small hilltop near the terminal where we spread out our materials and continued to work. Each of us independently arrived at the same conclusion: that Stephen Haines most likely died of natural causes and this was not a homicide.

The delay of the outgoing flight gave me the time to explain my findings on trace evidence and blood pattern evidence to Dr. Davis and Richard Kibbey. Trace evidence is often referred to as transfer evidence. This evidence is created by mutual transfer across the board when two surfaces come in contact. I had noticed gray-colored paint chips, various fibers, medium-velocity blood spatters, and rebound satellite spatters (blood drops falling into blood, causing a spatter resembling a satellite effect) on Stephen Haines's feet. These suggested that he was able to walk around his house and the garage with his bare feet. When his feet stepped into his own blood, he caused the blood transfer. His feet subsequently picked up the paint chips from the garage floor and fibers from the carpet in the house. If he was knocked down to the floor and was then beaten to death, then his feet would most likely be free of this trace evidence. The amount of paint chips and fibers and other trace evidence clearly indicated that he was, in fact, walking around the house for a long time before he collapsed on the garage floor. A closer study of the blood drops at the scene further revealed an interesting but very important finding. There were approximately four thousand to five thousand blood drops deposited on the kitchen, living room, bathroom, hallway, and garage floors. At least 60 percent of these blood drops were hollow/ghost-shape blood drops, meaning that the blood drop caused only a peripheral deposit but had no center. To observe this point, please see the samples below:

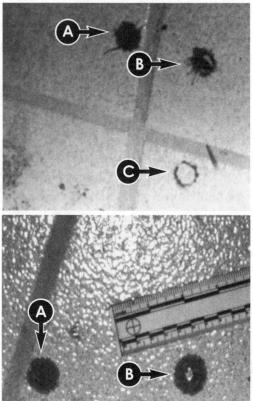

Three drops of blood were found on the living-room floor of the crime scene.
A represents a typical regular blood drop.
B shows a drop of blood mixed with some air.
C represents a hollow blood drop.

Close-up view shows two drops of blood on another section of the floor. Both of these drops originated from the same height.
A is a regular blood drop.
B is a hollow blood drop.

During the past forty-five years in my career as a police investigator and forensic scientist, I have had several experiences at crime scenes with these types of hollow/ghost blood drops. This type of blood drop is produced by vomiting or the coughing up of blood from the lungs. When liquid blood comes out of the mouth from the lungs or the trachea, this blood mixes with a large quantity of air bubbles. Once the blood is deposited on the surface where it is found, the air bubbles will most likely stay in the center of the blood drop. When the blood dries, the air bubbles will gush out and leave a ghost/hollow blood drop pattern. I remember about thirty years ago, I was called to a scene to assist in the investigation of a "homicide." When I arrived at the crime scene, the local police chief informed me that an elderly lady had been killed by her husband. I saw a man, motionless and without any expression, sitting in a rocking chair, covered with blood. The chief said it sure looked like he was guilty. That was until I examined the decedent's body and did not find any open wounds. However, the kitchen counter, table, and floor all were covered with blood drops—hollow/ghost drops—similar to the blood drops found in the bathroom. Large amounts of empty wine and liquor bottles were found all over the elderly couple's house. Then I noted that chronic alcoholism (a pathological condition resulting from the habitual use of alcohol in excessive amounts) often resulted in liver damage and the vomiting up of blood.

THE BARRATT HEARING

I arrived at the West Palm Beach Airport in the early afternoon of Sunday, July 30, to prepare my findings for a deposition scheduled for the following day at the Martin County Courthouse. This testimony would provide a scientific analysis that would back the defense's contention that Stephen Haines had died of natural causes and was not the victim of a homicide. Kibbey met me at the airport, and the two of us continued to go over the case's facts and my findings until midnight. The next day, I put on the record my determination that the trace blood pattern evidence found in the victim's home was not the result of a homicide, but was, instead, blood smearing consistent with a man drunk and struggling to move about his home. Under cross-examination by the prosecution, I testified that there was a large amount of blood present. I also said that, in contrast to Suzan Barratt's contention that Haines was a hemophiliac, he suffered from a thin blood condition due to his blood's containing a high percentage of alcohol. In making those assessments, I also relied on Haines's medical record from the hospital and the analysis provided by Dr. Joseph Davis.

Following my testimony, Richard Kibbey and I were confronted by the local media on the courthouse's steps, where we answered questions. I took this occasion to stress that "my position is not in favor of the defense or the prosecution, but to relate the scientific facts of the case." With that being said, I told the media that I did not feel that Stephen Haines was murdered. The following evening, Kibbey and his partner, Richard Barlow, hosted a reception on Hutchinson Island, where I gave a three-hour lecture and training seminar for local law enforcement officers, detectives, prosecutors, defense lawyers, and judges. More than two hundred people were in attendance. During my presentation, I shared with this select audience what I considered to be important concepts in the science of forensic investigation and crime scene reconstruction. In brief, I used case illustrations to show the procedures for a proper crime scene search and the steps that have to be taken to achieve an accurate and successful crime scene analysis.

In addition, I also pointed out the most fundamental issues of criminal investigations. It is most essential that the police investigator and forensic scientist keep an open mind in any case being examined. Detectives and forensic scientists have collected all the available information (both insculpatory and exculpatory) from the crime scene and the physical evidence. The major steps I explained in collecting this data and information involve the following: recognition, documentation, collection, preservation, examination, evaluation, interpretation, and reconstruction.

These eight major steps are central dogma for any investigation.

The investigators should follow all steps with standard and established protocols to make sure all the forensic evidence has been properly collected, examined, and evaluated. Whether for the police investigator or the forensic scientist, all of the goals are the same: providing the scientific facts to a court of law. These processes seem simple and straightforward. However, in practice, these processes represent quite a challenge. In fact, most of the time, when a case is being investigated, each and every one often has his or her own opinion (or theory) on the case. However, most of the general public's opinions (or theories) are based on the news media's accounts of the case, or are solely related to the opinions of midnight talk-show hosts or guest commentators. Very few individuals really know the true facts and account of the case. The so-called public opinion will sometimes develop a pretrial verdict. A person's guilt or innocence has at times been determined by the news media. That is why pretrial publicity has become a major concern and so often can adversely affect the outcome of a case. The pressure from the media, other investigators, the victim's/defendant's families and friends, and the authorities often is too great for younger investigative/forensic scientists to bear. Peer pressure and professional jealousies can especially prevent the forensic scientist from testifying on behalf of the defense. The media and establishment often portray the defense's forensic expert as a hired gun or a whore. Many times, because of this trend, there is a lack of quality representation for a defendant by a highly qualified defense attorney or forensic expert. Therefore, innocent individuals get convicted. In recent years, attorneys Barry Scheck and Peter Neufeld have helped to combat this alarming trend through the formation of their Innocence Project organization. Through this innovative body, they review those glaring questions, inconsistencies, and errors. Up to now, approximately 140 falsely convicted individuals, many even on death row, have been set free.

Florida Circuit Judge Robert Makemson convened the case's preliminary hearing in later August, and a trial date was tentatively set for October 23. On Friday, August 25, Richard Kibbey argued that a confession of an assault by Suzan Barratt on Stephen Haines to homicide detectives had been unfairly coerced out of her during their four-hour, secretly taped interview of the suspect shortly after Haines's body was discovered. Richard Kibbey made a motion to rule out any of the evidence gathered by police during the interview, as well as any evidence of bloodstains found on Barratt's clothing seized by the police. The prosecution argued that Barratt had willingly given her statements to the detectives and was given the opportunity to leave at any time. The police, however, admitted that a distraught Suzan Barratt had asked whether or not she needed an attorney but was not eager to get up and leave. The investigators also said that Barratt did not appear intoxicated during the interview, even though a blood sample taken two hours into the session indicated a blood/alcohol content of .024, which is three times the level at which a driver is presumed drunk. At one point, a detective pointed out a moment during the taped interview when he reminded Barratt that she had not been arrested and was free to leave at any time, if that was her choice. The detectives also testified that they offered Suzan Barratt beverages and let her smoke outside the station house, accompanied by her mother, Elaine Barratt.

During his cross-examination of the police investigators, Richard Kibbey hammered away at their failure to provide Suzan Barratt with any *Miranda* warning, as noted earlier: that she could remain silent, that anything she said could be held against her, and that she had the right to an attorney. Kibbey argued that the investigators, without an arrest and *Miranda* warning, felt they could continue this "noncustodial interview" for as long as they desired, in a clear violation of Suzan Barratt's rights. Mrs. Elaine Barratt also took the stand and testified that when her daughter had phoned her the morning after she'd found Haines's body, Suzan had been screaming and crying hysterically. Mrs. Barratt had accompanied Suzan to police headquarters and was present for portions of the police interview. Mrs. Barratt said that her daughter had seemed to wilt during the questioning, yet the two did not choose to leave police headquarters since they considered that an inappropriate thing to do. She also testified that the police had never read her daughter her *Miranda* rights, and she was never allowed to make a phone call.

On Friday, September 15, Judge Makemson announced his ruling that any and all statements made by Suzan Barratt during the four-hour police interview of October 4, 1999, could not be admitted into evidence in this case, because the interview had been conducted in a coercive manner. A member of the prosecution team later testified that the police had made statements to Barratt that indicated she was not free to leave any time she wanted. This was particularly so when a detective ordered her to stay in a police car in front of her home, when she was picked up and then taken to police headquarters, and when she was told to wait for questioning after she arrived at the station. The court also relied on my testimony that, in my opinion, Stephen Haines had died of natural causes, that the death most likely resulted from his being inebriated, his incurring multiple contusions, and the preexisting blood problem caused by his alcoholism.

On Thursday, September 22, the prosecution announced that it was planning to drop the second-degree manslaughter charge against Suzan Barratt for lack of evidence. Prosecutors also said that, in addition to the confession obtained in the tainted interview the day that Stephen Haines's body was found, any blood evidence scraped from Barratt's fingernails, the test of her own blood, and the blood evidence found on her clothing would all have been thrown out by the court.

THE SUMMARY

Following the decision to drop charges against Suzan Barratt, Richard Kibbey said that the mistakes the Port St. Lucie police investigators had made were due, in large part, to their inexperience. "They are a young department," Richard Kibbey explained. I respect this statement. We all make mistakes. When police investigators were looking about the garage in Suzan Barratt's and Stephen Haines's home and then at the blood smears in different rooms in this house, they jumped to a conclusion. This viewpoint only hardened with the coroner's conclusion that Haines had been the victim of a homicide.

Early on someone on the prosecution's side of the equation should have asked if, as an alcoholic, Stephen Haines might have died of natural causes. This would have saved Suzan Barratt and her family a great deal of anguish. And there was the danger that an innocent woman would have been found guilty of a crime she did not commit and sent to jail for a good many years. Our legal system is designed to protect the innocent, while prosecuting and punishing the guilty. As a component of the human equation, this justice system is not perfect, but it is the best that we can do.

Forensic evidence, I am proud to say, played a critical role in the proper resolution of this case. The scientific facts do not distort the truth. Rather, these facts present the truth. As I said when I arrived in Stuart, Florida, to testify on this case, the forensic evidence is never on one side or the other. Forensic evidence is only about the truth.

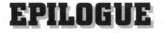

EPILOGUE

*Experience is a wonderful thing, when you find out
that you have made the same mistake again.*

—Dr. Henry C. Lee,
at several crime scenes

Even though I had my tongue in my cheek when I first uttered the statement above, rest assured I do not find any humor when I note that individuals assigned to a criminal investigation have made the same classic mistakes yet again. I usually just shake my head and report what I have seen to the individual who has asked me to work on a particular case. These mistakes are usually of a very rudimentary nature. Officers arriving at the Ramsey household at dawn the morning after Christmas are told JonBenet Ramsey has been kidnapped. They are then shown a ransom note, one that appears strange at face value. For seven hours the victim's body lies in a dark room behind the boiler in the family's basement. Finally,

John Ramsey and his best friend find the six-year-old's corpse. Everyone wants to solve this case, but how?

Mistakes. Crime scenes being contaminated. Bloodstain evidence not properly collected or correctly interpreted. A rush to judgment about a homicide when the dead man was a staggering alcoholic. It is true, as my words starting this chapter suggest, that it's easier to get over a mistake if it's not being made for the first time. But we must learn from our mistakes, a process that can begin once we acknowledge them. And we must vow not to repeat them. And, especially, an investigator should not develop tunnel vision on a specific case. Instead, he or she should always keep an open mind and let only the evidence lead to the case's solution.

Fortunately for all Americans, police work here is improving very steadily. Officers are increasingly well educated when they join the force, and in-service training has taken police investigative proficiency to new and higher levels. The National Institute of Justice has recognized the importance of crime scene investigation and has established a National Crime Scene Technology Center at the Henry C. Lee Institute of Forensic Science, the University of New Haven, to train forensic scientists and crime scene investigators from around the country. Meanwhile, DNA and other scientific breakthroughs have equipped investigators with amazingly accurate tools. Still, it is most essential that this forensic evidence be placed in its proper context. The wrongful jailing of five young men as rapists after the Central Park jogging assault of the early nineties stands as a historic warning to investigators to heed the context of the DNA evidence. Five assailants were imprisoned for a brutal physical and sexual assault, yet only one source of DNA was found, and this did not match any of the accused. How did this happen? Did the others use condoms? If it weren't for the true assailant's confession, these young men would still be in prison today.

I hope that the five case studies presented here have shed light on the complex challenges that confront the police officer and the forensic scientist. I have tried to break down the established facts underlying each crime into what William Shakespeare called "an hour glass of time." I will continue to pursue scientific facts, when and where I am asked to do so. I admit that I find this work fascinating, though at times depressing. I am most satisfied when I see the police, the prosecution, the courts, the media, and the public at large all cooperating to bring the guilty to justice and to free the innocent, clearing them of any blame for a crime. This is my life's work. I hope to pursue these duties for as many more years as God and my continued good health provide me. Perhaps someday soon, the enormous technological progress we have made in the forensic sciences field will mean that potential perpetrators will think twice before committing a ghastly crime. That way, we can all live in peace.

JONBENET RAMSEY RANSOM NOTE

Mr. Ramsey,

Listen carefully! We are a group of individuals that represent a small foreign faction. We respect your bussiness [*sic*] but not the country that it serves. At this time we have your daughter in our possession. She is safe and unharmed and if you want her to see 1997, you must follow our instructions to the letter.

You will withdraw $118,000.00 from your account. $100,000 will be in $100 bills and the remaining $18,000 in $20 bills. Make sure that you bring an adequate size attache to the bank. When you get home you will put the money in a brown paper bag. I will call you between 8 and 10 am tomorrow to instruct you on delivery. The delivery will be exhausting so I advise you to be rested. If we monitor you getting the money early, we might call you early to arrange an earlier delivery of the money and hence a [sic] earlier delivery [*delivery is subsequently crossed out*] pick-up of your daughter.

Any deviation of my instructions will result in the immediate execution of your daughter. You will also be denied her remains for proper burial. The two gentlemen watching over your daughter do not particularly like you so I advise you not to provoke them. Speaking to anyone about your situation, such as Police, F. B. I., etc., will result in your daughter being beheaded. If we catch you talking to a stray dog, she dies. If you alert bank authorities, she dies. If the money is in any way marked or tampered with, she dies. You will be scanned for electronic devices and if any are found, she dies. You can try to deceive us but be warned that we are familiar with Law enforcement countermeasures and tactics. You stand a 99% chance of killing your daughter if you try to outsmart us. Follow our instructions and you stand a 100% chance of getting her back. You and your family are under constant scrutiny as well as the authorities. Don't try to grow a brain John. You are not the only fat cat around so don't think that killing will be difficult. Don't underestimate us John. Use that good southern common sense of yours. It is up to you now John!

Victory!
S.B.T.C.

This note was printed by hand on three pages of 8½ × 11 inch white, lined stationery.

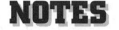

NOTES

CHAPTER ONE. THE CONCETTA "PENNEY" SERRA CASE: A FATHER'S QUEST

1. Paid advertisement, *New Haven Register*, July 16, 1988, p. 11.

2. Joseph Brady, "Unsolved 1973 Serra Murder Still Haunts New Haven," *New Haven Register*, September 24, 1989.

3. *The Crossroads, 1971*, Wilbur Cross High School Yearbook, New Haven, CT.

4. Robert A. Phillips, "Golino Arrested for Serra Murder," *New Haven Register*, July 6, 1984.

5. Nick Povenelli, "Ex-Wife Says Golino Threatened Her with Serra Killing," *New Haven Register*, September 24, 1989.

6. Ibid.

7. Ibid.

8. Ibid.

9. Christa Lee Rock, "Serra Murder Trial Opens," *New Haven Register*, April 30, 2002.

10. Christa Lee Rock, "Model Recreates Scene of '73 Serra Murder," *New Haven Register*, May 24, 2002.

11. Christa Lee Rock, "Prosecution Presents Blood Evidence in Serra Trial," *New Haven Register*, May 8, 2002.

12. Christa Lee Rock, "Yale Geneticist Raises Odds on Blood Only Being Grant's," *New Haven Register*, May 10, 2002.

13. Christopher Keating, "Focus on DNA Match," *Hartford Courant*, May 10, 2002.

14. Rock, "Yale Geneticist Raises Odds."

15. William Kaempffer, "More Proof Blood at Scene Was Grant's," *New Haven Register*, May 11, 2002.

16. Ibid.

17. Christa Lee Rock, "1973 Photo of Grant Takes Center Stage, Face of a Murderer?" *New Haven Register*, May 14, 2002.

18. Christa Lee Rock, "Prosecution Rests in Serra Case—No Motive Offered," *New Haven Register*, May 15, 2002.

19. Christa Lee Rock, "Emotional Time—Jurors Tour Crime Scene," *New Haven Register*, May 17, 2002.

20. Christa Lee Rock, "Undies Revealed Male DNA Traces," *New Haven Register*, May 21, 2002.

21. Ibid.

22. Ibid.

23. Christa Lee Rock, "Serra Case Nears End; Long Wait May Follow," *New Haven Register*, May 22, 2002.

24. Christa Lee Rock, "Serra May Have Fought to Protect Car, State Says," *New Haven Register*, May 23, 2002.

25. Ibid.

26. Christa Lee Rock, "Serra Jury to Resume Deliberations," *New Haven Register*, May 25, 2002.

27. Christa Lee Rock, "Guilty—Jury Convicts Grant of Murdering Penney Serra," *New Haven Register*, May 29, 2002.

28. Michelle Tuccitto, "Golino Still Insists Grant Innocent," *New Haven Register*, May 29, 2002.

29. Rock, "Guilty."

30. Michelle Tuccitto, "20-to-Life—Grant Sentenced in Penney Serra Murder," *New Haven Register*, September 28, 2002.

31. Josh Kovner, "Sentencing Ends 1973 Serra Case," *Hartford Courant*, September 28, 2002.

CHAPTER TWO. THE SKAKEL-MOXLEY CASE: A MURDER ON MISCHIEF NIGHT

1. Timothy Dumas, *Greentown: Murder and Mystery in Greenwich, America's Wealthiest Community* (New York: Little, Brown and Company, 1998), p. 23.
2. Ibid., p. 132.
3. Ibid., pp. 65–66.
4. Ibid., pp. 138–39.
5. Ibid., pp. 127–37.
6. Ibid., p. 137.
7. Ibid., pp.132–33.
8. Ibid., pp. 90–91.
9. Ibid., pp. 14–15.
10. Ibid., p. 16.
11. Ibid., pp. 31–32.
12. Ibid., p. 37.
13. Ibid., pp. 45–46.
14. Ibid., p. 51.
15. Ibid. pp. 19–20.
16. Mark Fuhrman, *Murder in Greenwich: Who Killed Martha Moxley?* (New York: HarperCollins, 1999), pp. 102–105.
17. Ibid., pp. 104–105.
18. Ibid., pp. 106–107.
19. Dumas, *Greentown*, pp.56–59.
20. Ibid., p. 153.
21. Ibid., pp.149–56.
22. Ibid., pp. 169–76.
23. Ibid., p. 180.
24. Ibid., p. 243.
25. Ibid., p. 222.
26. Ibid., pp. 252–54.
27. Ibid., pp. 229–31.
28. Ibid., pp. 224–29.
29. Ibid., pp. 243–44.
30. Ibid., pp. 244–48.
31. Fuhrman, *Murder in Greenwich*, p. 264.
32. Dumas, *Greentown*, pp. 247–48.
33. Ibid., pp. 268–72.

34. Ibid., p. 265.

35. Fuhrman, *Murder in Greenwich*, p. 158.

36. Ibid., pp. 96–112.

37. Rachel Gottlieb, "After Fighting Subpoena, Elderly Man Speaks Privately to Grand Juror," *Hartford Courant*, September 10, 1999.

38. Lynn Touhy, "Skakel Defense Faces Tough Fight on Two Fronts," *Hartford Courant*, June 28, 2000.

39. Ibid.

40. Michael Gannon, "Skakel Trial Opens With . . . Chilling Testimony," *New Haven Register*, May 8, 2002.

41. Ibid.

42. Michael Gannon, "Time Uncertain on Moxley Death, Experts Say," *New Haven Register*, May 9, 2002.

43. Peter Brooks, *Troubling Confessions: Speaking Guilt in Law and Literature* (Chicago: University of Chicago Press, 2000), pp. 8–33.

CHAPTER THREE. THE JONBENET RAMSEY CASE: A CRY IN THE NIGHT

1. Lawrence Schiller, *Perfect Murder, Perfect Town: JonBenet and the City of Boulder* (New York: HarperCollins, 1999), pp. 64–65.

2. Linda Edison McClean, *JonBenet's Mother: The Tragedy and the Truth!* (Parsons, WV: McClain, 1998), pp. 48–49.

3. Richard Jerome, "Mystery Couple," *People*, October 6, 1997, pp. 98–106.

4. Ibid.

5. Schiller, *Perfect Murder*, pp. 3–5.

6. Jerome, "Mystery Couple."

7. Schiller, *Perfect Murder*, p. 11.

8. Ibid., p.13.

9. Ibid., pp. 24–25.

10. Ibid., pp. 49–50.

11. Ibid., p. 50.

12. Ibid., p. 63.

13. Ibid., pp.65–66.

14. Ibid., p. 67.

15. Ibid., p. 79.

16. Ibid., pp. 89–90.

17. Ibid., pp. 90–91.
18. Ibid., pp. 172–76.
19. Ibid., p. 305.
20. Ibid., p. 302.
21. Ibid., p 316.
22. Ibid., p.358.
23. Ibid., pp. 368–69.
24. Ibid. p.384.
25. Ibid., pp. 386–87.
26. Ibid., pp. 388–89.
27. Ibid., p, 404.
28. Ibid., p. 425.
29. Ibid., p.463.
30. Ibid., p. 511.
31. Ibid., pp.535–37.
32. Ibid., pp. 547–50.

CHAPTER FOUR. THE LISA PENG CASE: ADULTERY AND DEATH

1. Qi Sing Wu, *Who Killed Jennifer Ji?* (Los Angeles: Lee Po Design & Productions, 1999), pp. 48–51.
2. Ibid., p. 71.
3. Ibid., p. 83.
4. Ibid., p. 46.
5. Ibid., p. 112.
6. Ibid., p. 99.
7. Ibid., p. 121.
8. Ibid., p. 77.

BIBLIOGRAPHY

Alcamo, I. Edward. *Biology* 2nd ed. Lincoln, NE: Cliffs Notes, 1995.

Asimov, Isaac. *The Genetic Code*. New York: Orion, 1962.

Baden, Michael, and Marion Roach. *Dead Reckoning: The New Science of Catching Killers*. New York: Simon & Schuster, 2000.

Bolsover, Stephen R., Jeremy S. Hyams, Steve Jones, Elizabeth A. Shepherd, and Hugh A. White. *From Genes to Cells*. New York: Wiley Liss, 1997.

Bosco, Joseph A. *A Problem of Evidence: How the Prosecution Freed O. J. Simpson*. New York: William Morrow, 1996.

Brooks, Peter, *Troubling Confessions, Speaking Guilt in Law and Literature*. Chicago: University of Chicago Press, 2000.

Connors, Edward, Thomas Lundegran, Neal Miller, and Tom McEwen. *Convicted by juries, Exonerated by Science: Case Studies in the Use of DNA Evidence to Establish Innocence after Trial*. Washington, DC: US Department of Justice, 1996.

DeForest, Peter R., Robert Gaensslen, and Henry C. Lee. *Forensic Science: An Introduction to Criminalistics*. New York: McGraw-Hill, 1983.

DiMaio, Dominic J., and Vincent J. M. DiMaio. *Forensic Pathology*. Boca Raton, FL: CRC, 1999.

Dumas, Timothy. *Greentown: Murder and Mystery in Greenwich, America's Wealthiest Community.* New York: Arcade Publishing, 1998.

Fuhrman, Mark. *Murder in Greenwich: Who Killed Martha Moxley?* New York: HarperCollins, 1999.

Geberth, Vernon J. *Practical Homicide Investigation: Tactics, Procedures, and Forensic Techniques.* Boca Raton, FL: CRC, 1999.

Haglund, William D., and Marcella H. Sorg, eds. *Forensic Taphonomy: The Postmortem Fate of Human Remains.* Boca Raton, FL: CRC, 1997.

Lee, Henry C., and Robert Gaensslen. *Advances in Fingerprint Technology.* 2nd ed. Boca Raton, FL: CRC, 2001.

Lee, Henry C., and Howard A. Harris. *Physical Evidence in Forensic Science.* Tucson, AZ: Lawyers & Judges, 2000.

Lee, Henry C., Timothy Palmbach, and Marilyn Miller. *Henry Lee's Crime Scene Handbook.* San Diego: Academic Press, 2001.

McClean, Linda Edison. *JonBenet's Mother: The Tragedy and the Truth!* Parsons, WV: McClain, 1999.

Schiller, Lawrence. *Perfect Murder, Perfect Town: JonBenet and the City Boulder.* New York: HarperCollins, 1999.

Thomas, Steve, and Don Davis. *JONBENET: Inside the Ramsey Murder Investigation.* New York: St. Martin's Press, 2000.

Wecht, Cyril. *Grave Secrets: A Leading Forensic Expert Reveals the Startling Truth about O. J. Simpson, David Koresh, Vincent Foster, and Other Sensational Cases.* New York: Penguin, 1996.

INDEX

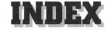

Asterisk (*) indicates use of a pseudonym